D0848118

THE
GOOD SCOTS DIET

THE

GOOD SCOTS DIET

What happened to it?

MAISIE STEVEN

ABERDEEN UNIVERSITY PRESS

First published 1985
Aberdeen University Press
A member of the Pergamon Group
© Maisie Steven 1985

The publisher acknowledges subsidy from the
Scottish Arts Council towards the publication
of this volume.

British Library Cataloguing in Publication Data

Steven, Maisie
  The good Scots diet: what happened to it?
  1. Food habits—Scotland—History
  1. Title
  641.3′009411   GT2853.G7

  ISBN 0-08-032429-0
  ISBN 0-08-032433-9 Pbk

PRINTED IN GREAT BRITAIN
THE UNIVERSITY PRESS
ABERDEEN

To remember Nan

CONTENTS

ILLUSTRATIONS

ACKNOWLEDGEMENTS

It would be difficult to acknowledge adequately all the help and encouragement I have received in writing this book. That it was ever begun at all is due to the inspiration of Mrs Joan Auld, archivist at Dundee University Library. Former Crieff librarians Roy and Andrene Flatt gave most generous assistance, at times even lending their personal books. I thank my friends Nannie Troup and Joan Macdonald warmly, not only for their typing skills but for much enthusiastic support besides. Warm thanks are also due to Mrs Morrison of Sidinish in South Uist, and to some elderly residents in my native Glen Urquhart, for sharing memories of food habits in their childhood.

In the decade of the 1790s, Sir John Sinclair of Caithness persuaded all the ministers of the Established Church of Scotland to respond to a list of 160 questions on every aspect of their parishes. The resultant *Statistical Account* has been of immense value in the writing of this present book, especially in providing a comparison between Highland and Lowland, urban and rural conditions.

For insights into world hunger I am greatly indebted to Tear Fund—an agency which we as a family are honoured to represent locally—as well as to Quaker family members Helen and Ellen. For all I have learned of Scotland's health problems, and also for much encouragement, I am most grateful to family friend and President of the McCarrison Society Dr Walter Yellowlees. Finally, to my husband Campbell I owe an incalculable debt for his always gently constructive criticism; while thanks are certainly due to our son Ken for his forbearance during a lengthy period of preoccupation—not to mention decidedly sub-standard nutrition on more than one occasion.

Sincere thanks are also due to the following authors and publishers for permission to quote from their works: Molly Weir and Hutchinson Books Ltd (*Shoes were for Sunday*); Dr Sandy Fenton, National Museum of Antiquities, Edinburgh (*Traditional*

Elements in the Diet of the Northern Isles of Scotland); Yehudi Menuhin and Macdonald and Co (Publishers) Ltd (*Unfinished Journey*); David Kerr Cameron and Gollancz (Victor) Ltd (*The Ballad and the Plough*), and the latter also for permission to quote from *Common Sense about a Starving World* by the late Professor Ritchie Calder; Tom Steel and The National Trust for Scotland (*The Life and Death of St Kilda*); Dorothy Hollingsworth, formerly director of the Nutrition Foundation (*A national Nutrition Policy: can we devise one?*); Bishop John V Taylor and S C M Press (*Enough is Enough*); Erik Dammann and Pergamon Press Ltd (*The Future in our Hands*); and Hodder and Stoughton Ltd for permission to quote from *The Prince in the Heather* by the late Eric Linklater.

Maisie Steven
Aberfeldy, Perthshire

PREFACE

This book began life as a 'short article'. Then the subject took over, and eventually some five years were spent in research and writing. During that time, several very different strands came to be woven into the final fabric.

The first was health. The study began at a time of much concern over Scotland's position in the league table for the 'diseases of civilisation', particularly for coronary heart disease. 'Western man', a leading article in the *British Medical Journal* had commented in the late seventies, 'has been lampooned as fat, toothless and constipated'. It looked then as if we Scots must be even fatter, more toothless and more constipated; and a growing number of health professionals were coming to see poor diet as a key contributory factor.

The next strand came from our past. It seemed natural to ask whether things had always been so bad, and to begin delving into Scotland's social history. The answer appeared to be no—certainly in the case of the rural population from the late eighteenth century onwards, subsisting on what could be called the traditional diet— although predictably, no clear overall pattern emerged. But both the early tourists and the parish ministers who penned the first two Statistical Accounts (for the 1790s, and 1835-45) were generally agreed that those rural Scots who had survived the undoubted hazards of childhood were remarkably healthy and vigorous. Surely, I began to think, the time must be ripe for a return to a simpler, more wholesome diet modelled on traditional patterns— though presumably with rather more modern appeal than an unremitting succession of broths and broses, potatoes and herring, neeps and kail.

Another strand was added through introduction to the McCarrison Society. I readily identified with the concern of this body of doctors, dentists and others over the potential effects upon health of an over-concentrated, refined diet, 'junk' foods and chemical additives; and with their belief in the vital role of good nutrition,

xi

and strong preference for wholesome foods grown on fertile soil. In researching the links between food and health, the renowned doctor/nutritionist Sir Robert McCarrison had, earlier this century, compared the dietary habits of different Indian races and had identified some who enjoyed outstandingly good health. It was exciting to realise that the diet of these people had practically everything in common with that of our own rural ancestors.

The fourth strand was a simple one—economy. Calculations revealed clearly that a simple diet of wholesome foods, although admittedly more costly in time and effort, was much cheaper than one relying heavily on processed items—an important point in view of rising unemployment.

The final strand seemed to lift the whole subject right out of the parochial into a world context, since what had happened to the Scots diet could serve as a warning in face of the erosion of traditional dietary practices in some developing countries today. But to my mind the most potent factor of all was the huge and seemingly ever-growing gulf between rich and poor countries. On the one side, gigantic food surpluses, wasteful food production, and a great deal of misery from diseases caused by overnutrition; on the other, desperate poverty, and a vast amount of misery from diseases caused by undernutrition. As Geoffrey Lean puts it in his book *Rich World: Poor World:* 'It is a situation which benefits nobody but the undertaker.'

1

THE EARLY CENTURIES

How was everybody fed?

In very earliest times, primitive man in Scotland must have had plenty of food—provided he was able to catch it.

The first men to reach our land—just how long ago is not known—would have been on the move, following the herds of animals, in Palaeolithic times when Scotland was joined to Ireland on the one side and Europe on the other. In *Scotland before History*[1] we read that in the region of 20,000 years ago

> man was already an old-established inhabitant of Europe, dependent for food and clothing on the animals with which he shared the arctic environment . . . following the herds of reindeer that were his main quarry as they moved over the tundra.

As, through many centuries, the ice-sheet gradually retreated and the habitable zone was extended, the 'food-gathering' Mesolithic peoples—their small seasonal settlements strung out mainly along the Atlantic coasts of the Hebrides and the western seaboard—were fishers as well as hunters and had a different kind of diet. Fascinating evidence of their countless fishy meals remains in the 'kitchen middens' composed of huge mounds of shells—whelks, limpets, cockles, oysters—found principally on the coast of Denmark but also to be seen in the West of Scotland. Remains of animal bones confirm, however, that the red and roe deer, the wild boar and even the seal formed part of their food as well.

The change from a hunting and food-gathering way of life to the profoundly different pattern of an agricultural economy is believed to have been made possible through the actual immigration of agricultural peoples. More than 5000 years ago, archaeologists tell us, the first agrarian colonists of the Neolithic Age reached our shores, bringing with them not only various seeds and plants, but domesticated animals as well.

1

Grain, both barley and wheat, had been known in the lands east of the Mediterranean from a very early period, so it is reasonable to suppose that it was from these countries that the knowledge of their cultivation stemmed. At first, it is probable that only small patches were cultivated, giving a quite inadequate yield of cereals, so that primitive man in Scotland continued as a hunter—of the elk and the red and roe deer, as well as of wild cattle and pigs.

A study of food refuse—not only of animal bones, but of charred grains and the impressions left by these upon pieces of pottery—can reveal much about ancient forms of domestic economy. Partly due to the warmer climate, Neolithic housewives had a more varied diet to set before their families than did their cave-dwelling predecessors—in all probability milk and curds, wild fruits, roots and nuts, in addition to the flesh of the deer and wild boar brought home by the men. Also, through using earthenware pots, they no longer needed to cook all their meat on spits over the fire, nor, using heated stones or embers, in pits dug in the ground. It was probably not until the latter part of the Neolithic period, however, that bread was made by grinding the corn, using a milling-stone and baking small loaves on a flat stone over the fire.

Turning to the Pictish people of Roman times, it is possible to piece together from archaeological findings some kind of picture of their domestic life. Of the 'wheel-house people' of the Outer Hebrides, colonists of the early Christian era, for example, T C Lethbridge in *The Painted Men* writes:

> These people were self-supporting farmers. . . . The evidence that they were great hunters, as well as herdsmen, agriculturalists and fishermen is very clearly shown in the South Uist and Benbecula wheel-houses. There are large quantities of red deer bones and many implements made from their antlers. . . . There are considerable numbers of bird-bones and also of sea-fish and seals. Whale bones are often found in the houses.[2]

It would thus be reasonable to suppose that these Pictish folk had quite a varied diet, the main part consisting of flesh, fish, and dairy foods. Exactly to what extent these would have been supplemented by cereals and various wild vegetables and fruits is difficult if not impossible to establish at this distance—how much easier if the vegetable kingdom left behind something as permanent as bones!

From early in the second millennium BC, we read, voyaging and trafficking went on between the folk of Scotland and Ireland, as well as with the southern parts of Britain and even as far afield as the Mediterranean, interchange that continued into historical times with the voyages of the Celtic saints. It is clear that trade with the South, by the land-routes through the Border passes as well as by coastal craft, was maintained from these early days onward. To piece together any kind of picture of domestic affairs in Scotland from this time until well into the mediaeval era is far from easy. Not only were a substantial number of deeds and chronicles either burned or removed by Edward I, but foreign writers rarely refer to domestic conditions in this country. One who does, however, is the French chronicler Froissart, who mentions that the French knights who came over in 1385 to march against England were appalled by the poverty they saw. The Feudal System was especially harmful to the poor in Scotland since, by the nature of the country, the nobles—remote from the Court and notoriously difficult to control—had an undue share of power: the common folk suffered accordingly.

It is to Froissart, too, that we owe interesting details of the character of border warfare. He describes the raiders' provisioning during their campaigns, including what must surely be the first description of the making of oatcakes:

> The Scots are bold, hardy and much inured to war. When they make their invasions into England they march from twenty to four-and-twenty miles without halting, as well by night as day. . . . They bring no carriages with them, on account of the mountains they have to pass in Northumberland: neither do they convey with them any provision of bread or wine, for their habits of sobriety are such in time of war that they will live a long time on flesh half-sodden, and drink the water of the river without wine. They have, therefore, no occasion for pots and pans, for they dress the flesh of their cattle in the skins; and, being sure to find plenty of cattle in the country which they invade, they carry none with them. Under the flap of the saddle each man carries a broad plate of metal; behind the saddle a little bag of oatmeal. When they have eaten too much of the sodden flesh, and their stomachs appear weak and empty, they place this plate over the fire, mix water with their oatmeal, and when the plate is heated, they put a little of the paste upon it, and make a thin cake like a biscuit, which they eat to warm their stomachs. It is, therefore, no wonder that they perform a longer day's march than other soldiers. In this manner the Scots entered England, destroying and burning everything as they passed.[3]

Scotland has always been a food-producing country, in spite of a climate not particularly conducive to the satisfactory ripening of field crops or, more especially, fruit. Until as recently as the late eighteenth century she could, at least in theory, produce enough food to feed her people. Although naturally it is difficult to estimate numbers in pre-census days, it is believed that the population was well below what the land could support, probably in the region of half a million; while even at the 1755 census it stood at only one and a quarter millions.

There is probably no such thing even today as a typical Scots diet. Certainly some people are far more nutrition-conscious than others; and some can afford to eat much more expensively than others. But on the whole the majority today can afford the basic foodstuffs required to keep them in reasonable health. Not so in mediaeval times. Generally speaking, the rich lived on the fat of the land while the poor ate frugally—or sometimes not at all.

Records tell us of recurrent dearths and even famines in Scotland. For example, in 1563: 'a year of dearth throughout Scotland . . . all things apperteining to the sustentation of man by triple and more exceeded their accustomed prices'. In 1577, 'ane great dearth of all kinds of victuals, through all Scotland, that the like was not seen in man's days afore'. And in 1595, a famine 'whereof was never heard tell of in any age before, nor ever read of since the world was made'.[4]

Attempts to form an accurate picture of the probable diet of the poorer folk in those times soon run into difficulties. While some records do exist—for example, in the Household Books of some of the great houses—exact calculations become virtually impossible: where payments in kind are made to servants, not only are the old Scots measures (probably in any case somewhat variable) hard to translate into modern terms, but it is also impossible to tell how many mouths they were expected to feed. Still, it seems likely that with daily allocations of such items as oat and barley bread, fowls, mutton, herrings, eggs and ale, many of those more sheltered workers in Scotland were faring not at all badly. In contrast, the lot of a large number of independent poorer people must have been altogether unenviable in times of dearth.

For the rich, the outlook was very different. John Knox was incensed at the kind of high living which French influence had introduced into Edinburgh in his time. A law was passed in 1581 which forbade 'superfluous banqueting'. Many writings make it clear that the upper classes feasted on a wide variety of meat, fish and game, enlivened by exotic imports such as foreign wines, fruits, preserves and spices.

The following description by the English poet John Taylor of his hospitable reception as a visitor to Scotland in 1618 probably provides a fair example of the food enjoyed by the nobility over a very considerable period.

I thank my good Lord Erskin, hee commanded that I always bee lodged in his lodging, the kitchen being always on the side of a bank, many kettles and pots boyling, and many spits turning and twisting, with great variety of cheeres; as venison baked, sodden, rost and stu'de beef, mutton, goates, kids, hares, fresh salmon, pidgeons, hens, capons, chickens, partridge, moore-coots, heathcocks, caperkellies, and tarmagants; good ale, sacke, white and claret, tent and most potent aquavitae.[5]

Some, in describing the life of the ordinary people of those times, have tended to paint an idyllic picture of a Scotland whose people were free to help themselves from an overflowing natural larder—fish from the lochs and rivers, wild game from the forests. Others have been more inclined to believe that this produce was enjoyed mainly by the landowners. They have stressed that while the common people of most countries were poor in mediaeval times, the poverty of the Scots was proverbial. The main reason was war—civil and religious wars, and continuous struggles with the old enemy, England. Much of the best agricultural land lay at the mercy of the English raiders.

As mediaeval times drew to a close, the bulk of Scotland's population were probably subsisting on a frugal diet comprising various 'broses'—made from the meal of barley, oats, beans and pease (split peas)—along with variable amounts of milk, butter and cheese; with fish as an addition in some areas. Broths were always popular, especially in the diet of the Highlanders. With the exception of those serving on large estates, whose 'hand-outs' have already been described, meat appears as a relatively rare item, being included only on festive occasions such as baptisms and marriages; while cultivation of vegetables seems to have been restricted almost entirely to the ubiquitous kail, every cottager eventually having his 'ain kail-yard'.

There is no doubt, however, that many wild vegetables eked out the meagre food supply—young nettles, wild garlic, sorrel, watercress; edible roots such as earthnuts and silverweed; and several varieties of seaweed in coastal districts. Hazel and beech nuts would have provided a welcome addition in autumn. Wild fruits too would have been eaten in season—brambles, blaeberries, cloudberries, raspberries.

Eggs are mentioned rarely; that they were considered important, however, is apparent from a Privy Council report referring to the year 1615:

> Amang the mony abuses whilk the iniquity of the time and private respect of filthy lucre and gain has produced within the commonwealth, there is of late discoverit a most unlawful and pernicious tred of transporting eggs furth of the kingdom. Certain avaritious and godless persons, void of modesty and discretion, preferring their awn private commodity to the commonweal, has gone and goes athort the country and buys the haill eggs that they can get, barrels the same, and transports them at their pleasure. There has been a great scarcity of eggs this while begane, and any that are to be had have risen to such extraordinar and heich prices as are not to be sufferit in a weel-governit commonwealth.[6]

Around the end of the seventeenth century the social history of Scotland makes particularly sad reading. From 1696 on, a series of seven seasons later known as 'the dark years', of practically year-long disastrous weather, caused an almost total failure of the crops, leading to unprecedented famine and misery. Writers have described the wretched state of the people, seen out in the fields in January and February vainly attempting to salvage some of the blackened, ruined grain. It is recorded that in some places one-third of the population died of starvation, while livestock perished in thousands. Bands of desperate folk prowled around the villages ready to fight for food; some are said to have even sold children in return for food; frequently people lacked the strength to bury their dead. Before the land had recovered from these lean years, another terrible famine came in 1709, bringing in its wake ruin for many farmers, as crops and cattle were destroyed wholesale. Many had to leave their land, much of which was not reclaimed for nearly a century. Henry Graham, in *The Social Life of Scotland in the Eighteenth Century*, gives a vivid account of those blackest of years:

> During these hungry years, as starvation stared the people in the face, the instincts of self-preservation over-powered all other feelings, and even natural affection became extinct in crowds of men and women forced to prowl and fight for their food like beasts. Old and young struggled together for the nettles, docks, and grass in spring, while they gathered greedily the loathed snails in summer and stored them for the winter's use.[7]

In his *Sketch of the Civil and Traditional History of Caithness from the Tenth Century* James T Calder gives an interesting picture of conditions in the North which had doubtless prevailed for centuries:

Before the introduction of potatoes, the diet of the lower classes was very poor, consisting generally of brose or porridge to breakfast, of cabbage boiled with a mixture of oatmeal for dinner, and of bere bread and brochan (water gruel) for supper. Butcher meat, with the exception of a little pork, rarely appeared at table. Sowens, when it was to be had, was a favourite dish for breakfast, dinner, or supper. Another favourite dish was 'bursten', which was prepared by a portion of oats and bere being hastily dried in a pot over the fire, and then ground in a hand-quern. The kind of meal thus produced, when taken with milk, formed a very palatable dish, and was by many preferred to the ordinary porridge. The inhabitants along the sea-coast, when fish was to be had, got on pretty well; but when they were prevented by rough weather from going to sea, or when, as sometimes happened, the fish appeared to have left the coast, they had recourse to shellfish, such as limpets, mussels, and periwinkles, which were but an indifferent substitute for the other. One luxury, however, they had which their descendants are deprived of, namely, good home-brewed ale.

The gentry, on the other hand, though without the refinements and luxuries of modern life, lived well and sumptuously. They had plenty of meat roasted and boiled, and abundance of wine, particularly claret; and when whisky punch became the order of the day, they did ample justice to it.[8]

The practice of bleeding cattle as a means of supplementing the human diet was well established in eighteenth-century Scotland, but doubtless originated long before. An entry in the *Statistical Account for Fortingall, Perthshire, refers to it thus:*

It is hardly possible to believe on how little the Highlanders formerly lived. They bled their cows several times a year, boiled the blood, ate a little of it, and a most lasting meal it was. The present incumbent has known a poor man, who had a small farm hard by him, by this means, with a boll of meal for every mouth of his family, pass the whole year.[9]

In his classic work *The Drove Roads of Scotland,* Dr A R B Haldane comments that drovers short of food may well have bled the cattle on their long, hard journeys to the trysts: 'The blood, with the oatmeal and onions which they carried, would supply the main ingredients for the black puddings, which were a traditional Scottish food.'[10]

In view of the undoubted privations suffered in times of scarcity, and indeed the frugality of the diet generally, it may come as something of a surprise that various visitors of the time write sometimes glowing accounts of the health of Scotland's folk. An Englishman called Chamberlayne, visiting Scotland early in the eighteenth century, observed that the diet of the Scots is agreeable to their estates and qualities. The tradesmen, farmers and common people are not excessive devourers of flesh, as men of the same rank are in England. Milk-meats and oatmeal, several ways prepared, and kail and roots dressed in several manners, is the constant diet of the poor people (for roast meat is seldom to be had but on gaudy-days); and with this kind of food they enjoy a better state of health than their southern neighbours, who fare higher.[11]

Captain Burt,[12] an Englishman who was General Wade's agent and surveyor in the North of Scotland during the 1720s, made some lengthy comments about the contemporary Highland scene: although these were not always complimentary, it has to be said that he comes across as a shrewd and accurate observer. He wrote much about the poverty of the Highland people, yet allowed that their health was generally good in view of the frugality of their food—mostly milk and oatmeal. 'They are very healthy and free from distempers', he comments, 'notwithstanding the great hardships they endure. I own they are not very subject to maladies occasioned by luxury.' Not surprisingly, the coin had another side: 'They are very liable to fluxes, agues, coughs, rheumatisms, and other distempers, incident to their way of living.' This accords with the impression one receives several decades later, from the resident contributors to the *Statistical Account*. Again and again we read that the people are 'remarkably healthy', and that 'the principal maladies are the rheumatism and sundry fevers'.

It seems clear that an adequate, if limited, diet was available to the poor in times of relative prosperity. When the crops failed for any reason, they faced want, or at times starvation. A study of the agriculture of the time provides the key to this situation. Henry Graham writes:

> Whenever seasons were bad and crops were blighted, the peasantry were always reduced to extremity. Years of dearth came often, and as in 1709, and 1740, and 1760, the condition of the people was woeful. If we ask why this was, and why such a disastrous state of the people occurred in Scotland, we find the explanation—not in the unpropitious northern climate, in its excess of rain, and mist, and cold—but in the barbarous mode of its agriculture.[13]

The run-rig system, whereby alternate strips of land were cultivated by different farmers, had much to answer for, since improvements such as drainage and enclosure were not possible; thus in winter the whole became a kind of common over which all the cattle wandered unchecked. A sad picture emerges of land largely unfertilised and undrained, often choked with weeds; of almost total ignorance of crop rotation, with arbitrary ideas of sowing dates, which frequently meant harvesting far too late; of antiquated, unwieldy implements, such as ploughs requiring up to a dozen oxen to draw them; of draught animals so weak and emaciated that it was not uncommon for neighbours to have to help each other to raise them to their feet. Cows were often so undernourished that they calved only every few years; and as no sown grasses, and no turnips, were being cultivated, a great many cattle had to be killed off before winter, being salted down for later use.

Added to this somewhat grim picture was the burden under which the common folk laboured in being obliged to give both work and produce in return for the use of the land; nor, indeed, could it be said that this system necessarily benefited the landlords either, because with rents paid in kind they had too little cash and far too many provisions (meal, fowls, eggs, cheese, butter) which must have led to much prodigality and waste.

A last but vital deterrent to any kind of prosperous rural economy lay in the widespread dearth of roads, and the parlous state of such as did exist. Many writings of the era make it abundantly clear that these were the bane of travellers to Scotland in those times. Graham says:

> In driest weather highways were unfit for carriages, and in wet weather were almost impassable even by horses—deep ruts of mire, covered with big stones, now winding up heights, now zigzagging down steep hills, to avoid the swamps and bogs.[14]

Again, nothing was a greater hindrance to any kind of marketing—even between one farm and another—than the lack of suitable conveyances. All produce had to be transported in sacks on horseback, or on sledges, with tumbling wheels of solid wood (known as tumbrils), or else, of course, on the backs of those other beasts of burden of the day—women. The cart did not come into general use until the 1760s. It is recorded in the *Statistical Account* that when, in 1723, a cart was used to carry a small load of coals from East Kilbride to Cambuslang, a large crowd went out to view this wonderful new contraption.[15] But even had there been carts before that date, it seems highly unlikely that the roads would have supported them.

In some areas the early efforts of some of the most worthy 'improvers' were baulked at every turn; new agricultural methods were spurned, and dykes and young hedges destroyed where attempts were being made to enclose the land. Superstition, bigotry and stubbornness all held sway, as did the tendency to ascribe all disasters to the will of God.

Even road-making met with surprisingly fierce opposition. Some lairds refused to have roads near their houses, nor would the tenantry suffer them near their farmhouses, because of a (probably well-founded) fear of being invaded by thieves and vagrants. One group of traders who did manage to carry on their business in spite of this were the cadgers (single-horse traffickers), well-known characters in Scotland right up to the nineteenth century. They carried fish, poultry, eggs, and probably much besides, and appear to have been equal to the roughest tracks of the day, as is suggested by the 'cadgers' yetts' (gates) which remain in some remote places to perpetuate their memory.

An excerpt from the *Statistical Account* for Cambuslang (written in 1790 but actually describing the state of the land there forty years previously) offers an interesting summary of the very conditions we have been considering:

> Most of the farms run-rig, that is, the lands of one farmer intermixed with those of another.
>
> The tenants bound to lead their landlords' coals, and to give him some days' work in seed-time and harvest.
>
> The roads narrow and rough, scarcely passable with carts in summer, and in winter so deep as to be hardly passable with horses.
>
> No wheat, no hay made of clover and rye grass, no potatoes planted in the fields.
>
> No wheat bread, no sugar and tea used, but by people of wealth and fashion, and not much by them.
>
> Little butcher meat consumed; no fat cattle killed, except by gentlemen, and some of the greatest farmers.[16]

Taken all in all, Scotland and her agriculture would certainly appear to have reached rock-bottom around this time. Fortunately, however, better things were already on the horizon—nearer, indeed, than anyone could have dreamed. By the following century such a complete reversal had taken place that Scottish agriculture was actually being held up to the old rival, England, as a shining example.

2

THE BEGINNINGS OF IMPROVEMENT

What changed the scene?

The Jacobite Risings; the Napoleonic Wars; the Turnpike Act of 1751; smallpox vaccination; the turnip and the potato. Surely a strangely assorted list with no very obvious common denominator. Yet in the quite remarkable advances in agriculture and social life which characterised the latter half of the eighteenth century in Scotland, each of these played such a significant part that it is of interest to look at them briefly as part of the background to the dietary study.

Despite a bief aura of glory and romance, the Jacobite Risings of 1715 and 1745 brought a great deal of hardship to the Highland people. Yet one blessing followed in their wake—the new roads which opened up access and facilitated trade between the Lowlands and Highlands. Despite the levying of tolls which in some areas had been introduced in 1714, the Turnpike Act of 1751 represented by far the most significant step forward towards the urgently needed road improvements: for example, the fact that the heavy coach which ran between Edinburgh and Glasgow, taking twelve hours for the journey in the mid eighteenth century, had reduced this time to five hours by the early nineteenth century, shows just how greatly communications had improved during that period.

A small entry in the *Statistical Account* for Lochwinnoch, Ayrshire, in 1792 sums up neatly what must have been happening all over the country at the time:

> The roads were some years ago in a wretched state, hilly, narrow, and almost impassable in wet weather; but many of them are now excellent, and great improvements may immediately be expected, from two lines of new turn-pike road.[1]

It is therefore not surprising that by the end of the eighteenth century the marketing of food surpluses in the fast-growing centres of population was at last becoming possible, and at a mere fraction

11

of the former cost. It may be added that, had this not been so, the Industrial Revolution would not have been possible.

As for the Napoleonic Wars, their main effect would seem to have been to arouse in Scottish hearts a patriotic determination to increase food production by reclaiming and cultivating every possible acre of land. The demand for beef was greatly increased during this time, something which could be said to have begun to lay the foundations of the future fame of Scotch beef. Perhaps profiting most from the soaring price of beef were Scotland's drovers, one of whom is said to have remarked as he heard the bells ring out in 1815, that the peace would cost him dear.

On the public health scene, too, progress was at last beginning to gain momentum. Much emphasis is rightly given by social historians to the arrival, in the late eighteenth and early nineteenth centuries, of the smallpox vaccine. Along with water-borne typhoid and insect-borne plague, smallpox had been one of the truly devastating diseases prevalent in Scotland; and it is clear that vaccination represented a vital advance in preventive medicine which was to play its part in an unprecedented population increase—from something over a million in 1700 to nearly three million in 1855. The *Statistical Account* sheds valuable light on the scene, particularly as regards the resistance of the common folk in many areas to the new prophylactic technique. Let us hope that the worthy minister who penned the East Kilbride report exaggerated to some extent when he wrote:

> The smallpox sometimes rages with great fury. Inoculation, the best remedy for that mortal contagion, meets here with a bad reception. Rooted prejudices, founded upon arguments, some of which are trifling, and others absurd, influence the minds of the people so much against it, that they sit still, in sullen contentment, and see their children cut off in multitudes.[2]

Fortunately these prejudices do not seem to have extended to all areas. In Blackford (Perthshire), the writer was able to report:

> Formerly the smallpox never appeared in the parish without proving fatal to one out of every three whom they seized. But the country people have been taught to change their way of managing children in that disease; and some are so hardy as to inoculate their children with their own hand, so that very few die of that distemper.[3]

In the previous chapter, we looked at the Scotland of the early eighteenth century, a land which appeared to have reached such an all-time low that many must have despaired of ever seeing better times. We saw an agricultural system bedevilled by malpractice and ignorance, and a people living, at least in bad years, under threat of want or even famine. Yet within the brief space of about half a century, altogether undreamed-of improvements had been achieved. Naturally these were much slower to arrive in some places—for the most part in the remote areas of the Highlands and Islands—and, as must always happen, the 'improvers', mainly landed proprietors and some of the wealthier farmers, were well ahead of the general thinking of the time and often had to suffer misunderstanding and even abuse. But once the efficacy of the new methods began to be recognised, the trickle became a stream and there was no stopping it.

The extent to which the Union with England in 1707 contributed to Scotland's improved economy is something on which Scots historians are not entirely in agreement. While some tend to expatiate upon the poverty prevailing in Scotland at the beginning of the eighteenth century, others have hotly denied it, pointing out that not only are the beginnings of a forward movement evident in the previous century, but also that Scotland by no means slavishly followed her southern neighbour in every respect. Be this as it may (and surely poverty is in itself no cause for shame, except in so far as its cause may lie in bigotry or ignorance, or in the greed of a minority) it should surely be allowed that the closer trading links, and development in many ways following the pattern set by England, did indeed play a significant part in bringing about the profound improvements of the latter half of the century.

It may seem like wild exaggeration to say that the introduction of the turnip heralded the Agricultural Revolution, but this does certainly seem to be true. Up to this time, it had been the custom because of lack of winter feeding to slaughter most of the cattle at Martinmas, and to salt the meat (known in Scotland as the 'mart') for payment of rent and occasional winter use. All this and much more changed when the turnip—previously cultivated in the gardens of the rich, and used by them chiefly as a dessert—became a field crop. Here at last was good winter feeding for livestock, leading in turn to the possibility of improved stock-breeding; here also a nourishing vegetable, and a much-needed source of vitamin C into the bargain, which would eventually come to add variety to the diet of the rural folk, as well as providing an addition to the small crop rotation of the time.

Large claims indeed for the humble turnip, a vegetable which has certainly fallen in the social scale today. What then of the potato?

The new root was introduced to Britain from Virginia in the seventeenth century, and before long had become popular in Ireland, where it was soon to become the staple of the people. It took longer, however, to be accepted in Scotland. It is estimated that by the 1770s it had reached all over the Highlands and Islands, in the diet of whose people it was to play a part which can scarcely be over-emphasised. Gradually it took its place alongside dairy produce and cereals as a mainstay of the diet. In a Perthshire (Little Dunkeld) report towards the end of the century we read:

> This root has proved more beneficial to the country than perhaps any production of the land, lint excepted. It has saved the tenants from the ruinous necessity of purchasing meal for their families to a prodigious amount. It is not above 22 years since potatoes were introduced into the field . . . yet this vegetable may be reckoned a full third of the food of the common people. They are as healthy and vigorous, at least, as before. By means of this root the produce of the parish is fully adequate to the maintenance of its inhabitants.[4]

It was in the far Northwest and in the Hebrides especially that potatoes were to mean quite literally the difference between life and death. Thomas Pennant, visiting Skye in 1772, made this observation:

> Bear [barley] and small oats are the common produce of Skie; but the land is too wet to ripen them to perfection; and the produce of the crops is very rarely in any degree proportioned to the wants of the inhabitants: the years of famine are as ten to one. The grand helps of bad years are potatoes; a root whose cultivation cannot be too earnestly recommended to the poor, in any country.[5]

But if we follow the history of the potato into the next century, we find an altogether less rosy picture. This was the troubled era of the Clearances, when the pattern of settlement was forcibly changed, the people having the choice either of emigrating or of setting up coastal townships and building a fishing industry, leaving the hilly inland areas free for the more lucrative sheep-rearing. During this hard time potatoes were being planted in every available patch of soil, sometimes literally in nooks and crannies between the rocks. It is estimated that potatoes comprised some 75 per cent of the Highlanders' and Islanders' diet, a potentially dangerous state of affairs, should fishing catches and potato crop fail simultaneously. And fail they sometimes did; notably in the mid 1840s, when Government intervention became necessary on account of famine conditions. Emigration—either abroad, or to the rapidly-growing cities of the South—was perforce the only course open to large numbers of starving people at that time.

Osgood Mackenzie of Gairloch in Ross-shire, writing of the famine at first hand—despite having been very young at the time—gives some perspective to that calamitous event: not least, the benevolent paternalism of some of the old Highland chiefs, which had long since died out by then in many other areas, becomes apparent. 'There were soon to be very trying times during the great famine caused by the potato blight,' he writes in *A Hundred Years in the Highlands*:

> I have quite clear recollections of being made to eat rice, which I detested, instead of potatoes, with my mutton or chicken in the years 1846-1848, for even *Uaislean an tigh mhòr* (the gentry of the big house) could not get enough potatoes to eat in those hard times. Certainly things looked very black in 1846-1848 in Ireland and the West of Scotland.[6]

He goes on to tell of his mother's plan to finance the building of much-needed roads in the district:

> With the help of Government and begging and borrowing (I think) £10,000, she and my uncle undertook the great responsibility of guaranteeing that no one would be allowed to starve on the property.

As a little boy he was allowed to cut the first turf of the new road:

> How well I remember it, surrounded by a huge crowd, many of them starving Skye men, for the famine was more sore in Skye and the islands than it was on our part of the mainland.

After the famine the potato ceased to be the main dietary staple, although it did continue as an important food as well as part of the wages of many farm servants. In some parts, too, the growing of potatoes gave rise to pig-rearing as an industry.

Returning, however, to the Scotland of the latter half of the eighteenth century, we find a steady, heartening betterment of social conditions, following upon some overdue agricultural advances. We see soil extensively drained, limed and manured; land everywhere being enclosed by walls and hedges; vital crop rotation beginning to be observed; widespread planting of trees. Very importantly too, we find the unwieldy ploughs giving place to smaller and infinitely more manageable models, and other improved implements making their appearance. Selected grasses were beginning to be grown for cattle fodder. There were in addition two beneficial changes with far-reaching results—the ending by Act of Parliament of the archaic run-rig system; and the gradual cessation of the practice of payment of rents in kind, leading naturally to a greater availability of cash to enable landlords to carry out necessary improvements.

The credit for these immense advances must be shared between many enlightened landowners and farmers and the various 'improving societies' of the time whose aim was the wider dissemination of knowledge, both of agriculture and of gardening. To these the great majority of landowners gave their support, since there was an acute awareness of the pressing necessity to emulate that husbandry which so clearly had freed Scotland's richer neighbour from the threat of famine. First in the field in 1723, following a period of great want, was a society with the impressive name of The Honourable the Society of Improvers in the Knowledge of Agriculture in Scotland, who proclaimed splendidly that they

> resolved to put their Hands to Work, and their Pens to Paper, and so to employ their strenuous Endeavours, both by Example and Direction, to promote the Improvement of their Country and raise the Spirit thereof to the greatest Height possible.

This fine society unfortunately died out, but not before it had made a decisive contribution to the contemporary scene. The Highland and Agricultural Society which followed in 1784, and the Caledonian Society in 1809, also deserve credit for the immense advances they made possible, not least in the realm of cottage gardening—leading eventually, of course, to a most beneficial increase in the variety of available foods.

All of these improvements added up to a very considerable increase in food production. Scotland had at last embarked upon an era of agricultural prosperity which was to continue unchecked until, towards the close of the nineteenth century, the arrival on the market of grain from the rich prairie lands of North America began to pose a serious threat to her cereal producers, particularly in the prosperous 'model' farming areas of the Lothians.

If ever there was an era of maximum change, it was surely the latter half of the eighteenth century. In reading the *Statistical Account* one cannot fail to catch something of the excitement of that last decade of the century, as writer after writer strives in his own way to depict the kind of changes which were beginning to bring new hope and promise to the ordinary folk of Scotland.

The writer of the *Statistical Account* for Dowally in Perthshire, clearly interested in improving agricultural methods, writes

It was not difficult for an enlightened observer to trace the causes which produced and had perpetuated the rude state of agricultural practice. Where there are burdensome services to be performed by the tenant; where there is no inclosing, and no winter feeding; where leases are short, and where the farm of one tenant consists of disconnected patches, lying interspersed with the patches of other tenants, it is impossible that in any case agriculture should advance in improvement. (The Highlander labours under other great disadvantages in this respect. Having little intercourse with the low country, he has few opportunities of seeing the improved modes of culture practised there; and even when he does casually see them, his ignorance of the language of the improver prevents his gaining any minute or beneficial acquaintance with them.) The new arrangements respecting the crops and the culture of the parish, drew their efficacy from the following rules:

1. That each tenant should have the fields of his farm contiguous to each other, and be encouraged to inclose them.
2. That all burdensome services should be abolished.
3. That sheep should be excluded from the low grounds in winter.
4. That leases of due length should be granted.
5. That a proper rotation of crops should be prescribed.[7]

That there were occasional exceptions to the general rule becomes apparent from this somewhat contemptuous entry for Glasford, Lanarkshire:

The spirit of improving land has not yet reached this parish. There is in it only one man who deserves the name of a farmer. To improve land requires both industry and skill. Few of the farmers here have a moderate portion of either and many are defective in both.[8]

Many writers, however, were emphatic in conveying the message of optimism, and the following report from a Perthshire parish (Clunie) seems to provide an admirable summary of all that we have just been examining in the Scottish rural scene:

It is only of late years that the knowledge of agriculture, and the spirit of improvement, began to display themselves in this parish . . . The lands were no where subdivided or inclosed, and the country being open in winter as well as in summer, all things were common, and men and beasts were at liberty to prey upon one another. Happily for the place, the pleasure and the advantage of the people, the scene has now assumed another and a better appearance. Commonties and runrigs are done away; each man begins to know his own, and to have it in his power to improve it. Wet grounds are drained; rough grounds are cleared; stone-fences are built, and hedges are planted . . . rich clays are applied to lands, and a good soil formed, where there was no soil before; green crops begin to be raised, and a regular rotation of crops begins in some places to be understood. Many new instruments of husbandry are now introduced; many old prejudices, that had long retarded the progress of improvement, are laid aside. In the course of the last 40 years, the rents are in most places doubled, and though in every respect the expense of living has more than kept up with the rise of the rents, it is a fact, that both the farmers and their families are better lodged, better dressed, and better fed than ever.[9]

3

THE RURAL PEOPLE'S DIET

What made it so good?

Our brief study of eighteenth century advances would cause us to assume that there was a gradual improvement in the lot of the rural folk—who still, it should be remembered, comprised the great majority of Scotland's population—and would thus lead us to expect that their diet had also undergone some improvement. And, for the most part, we find that this was so.

That their physique was generally of a high standard is attested not only by records showing the numbers of country men recruited to Guards regiments, but also by the comments of various visitors to Scotland—writers who frequently expressed sheer incredulity at the vigour and endurance of agricultural labourers able to sustain a working day which might well begin at the 'unsocial hour' of 4 or 5 am and continue to as late as 7 or 8 pm. In addition, they were clearly astonished that these feats were accomplished by people whom they considered to be quite inadequately fed.

While often making mention of the fevers which ravaged the people from time to time, the writers of the *Statistical Account* in the 1790s also stress the generally high standard of health, some indeed citing quite remarkable cases of longevity. Not at all unusual is the entry for Fortingall, in Perthshire:

> In general, the people are long-lived. Many are between 80 and 90; some between 90 and 100; a few live beyond that age. The present incumbent likewise knew, about 30 years ago, one D. C., who lived, it was credibly asserted, to the amazing age of 127.[1]

Not to be outdone, a neighbouring writer quotes the case of M. S., a farmer aged 103, who 'walked a journey of 26 miles in one day at the age of 97, without complaining of weariness'. Most reports, while claiming no unusual records, yet emphasise the people's health and vigour, a typical comment being: 'Although there are no remarkable cases of longevity, yet the people in general are remarkably healthy.'

We are surely entitled to suppose that the diet of those times, even if considered to be only one environmental factor, did contribute significantly to the health of our rural ancestors, and to enquire what was the nature of this frugal fare which enabled them to accomplish such feats of endurance. With remarkably little variation, theirs was to be the diet of the vast majority of Scottish rural folk for well over a century—even, in some remote parts, until well into the present century—as well as possessing the main characteristics associated in our minds with the traditional Scots diet.

It is difficult to make confident assertions about any typical diet from this distance, particularly as regards quantities: these would obviously vary according to season and prosperity. What we do know is that the mainstays were whole cereals and dairy foods. Clearly too there were regional variations—in some areas, notably the east coast and the Hebrides, more fish; in the Northern Isles, again more fish, and a considerable amount of barley; in the Highlands as a whole, more potatoes than turnips, and so on. What we can do is to make up a composite sample of the likely menu of a typical cottar family of the day.

The working day would begin early with a bowl of oatmeal brose or porridge, or a kind of gruel known as brochan, washed down with either milk or ale, and followed by oat or barley bannocks. Surprisingly to us, these would be eaten dry, since such little butter as was eaten was used almost exclusively in cooking or served with potatoes: the rest was mixed with tar and applied as an antiseptic and water-repellent to the coats of livestock. The noon meal— depending of course on season—might consist of potatoes in some form, possibly served whole with butter or in some kind of broth, and again accompanied by bannocks, and milk or ale. An alternative might be the peculiarly Scots dish called 'sowens' (see description in Chapter 4) or again porridge, while the ever-popular kail might well appear. And for supper there could be kail, turnip or cabbage, possibly with the juice incorporated along with meal in a kind of brose; or barley broth, once again with oat or barley cakes and a drink of milk or ale—this last progressively replaced by tea from about the mid eighteenth century onwards. Cheese, made in Scotland from early times, might well be included (probably in modest amounts) at one or another of the meals; James Boswell's observations suggest that this might often be at breakfast.

A brief pause at this point might be salutary, to allow our mental gaze to roam around the laden shelves of our local supermarket, recalling the plethora of attractive imported items which enliven our daily fare; and then to ask ourselves how we would feel about facing up to these meals day in, day out, year after year. Whether, however, we find ourselves describing our ancestors' food as plain but wholesome, monotonous or merely grim, the point of present interest is principally to look at the nutritional quality of the diet. What goodness did it possess which made the majority of Scots rural dwellers such a sturdy and vigorous race? The best way to find out is by attempting to reconstruct the basic daily intake of, say, a male agricultural worker, and to calculate its nutritional value. An estimate could be made as follows:

Foods	Weight oz	Protein g	K Calories	Calcium mg	Iron mg
Potatoes	20	8.0	460	24	2.8
Oatmeal	8	27.2	920	126	9.36
Kail	4	0.8	12	66	0.52
Turnips	4	0.8	12	62	0.4
Barley	2	4.4	204	6	0.38
Butter	1	—	226	4	0.05
Cheese	1	7.2	120	230	0.16
Milk	1 pint	18.0	380	680	0.4
Ale	1 pint	1.4	160	38	0.2
		67.8	2494	1236	14.27
DHSS recommendations (1979) for a very active man		84.0	3350	500	10.0

It should at once be pointed out that this list refers to basic daily foodstuffs only, and allows for no extras at all. Also, the amounts calculated are probably somewhat low, at least for times of relative plenty. Suppose the milk intake were increased to two pints, this would bring the protein total up from 68 g to 86 g, a very satisfactory level. (The recommended allowance for protein by FAO standards is in any case considerably lower). Oatmeal consumption, too, could easily have been more than 8 oz: allocations per day on some of the great estates were often 1 lb or more. As for potatoes, if it is borne in mind that Irish agricultural labourers could cope with several pounds daily, 20 oz does not seem unduly generous.

In the above estimate it is energy which is far too low for a hard-working man: doubling the allowance of milk, oatmeal and potatoes would, however, add some 1800 kcal, bringing the total to approximately 4300. Whisky could have been another energy source for some. Elizabeth Grant in her *Memoirs of a Highland Lady*[2] states that the men of Speyside were accustomed to drink three goblets per day: taking this as a half-pint, another 600 kcal could have been added.

It will be seen that the calcium total is high and that for iron satisfactory; while in a diet as unrefined as this one the important group of B vitamins will be well represented. As for the fibre content, it must surely speak for itself.

There are three potentially weak points in this otherwise very good diet. These, as in all predominantly cereal-based diets, are the deficiencies of the vitamins A, C, and D. Searching for possible sources of these is in fact quite a fascinating exercise. Vitamin C is of all the nutrients the most difficult to estimate. Because it is easily destroyed, it is not possible to choose an arbitrary amount of those foods known to contain it and calculate their values from a book. In our chosen menu, all the same, 20 oz of potatoes, 4 oz of kail and 4 oz of turnips should certainly have provided more than enough, no matter how long or how badly cooked by our standards. But what of those times when potatoes, and possibly kail and turnips as well, were scarce or unavailable? One cannot be certain whether the vital connection between scurvy prevention and vegetables had been made to any extent (if at all), nor do we know how much the people depended upon wild plants, such as nettles. In the *Statistical Account* for Clunie, Perthshire, the writer mentions, for example, the use of 'watercresses, sloes, hawthorns, hipthorns, wild rasps, hazelnuts, crab apples'.[3] Rosehips, our countryside's richest source of vitamin C, would unfortunately be ripe at the same time as the potato crop. That few oranges or lemons ever reached the rural folk we do know, although these had been imported from the fifteenth century onwards.

A remark made by James Boswell in his *Journal of a Tour to the Hebrides*[4] is of interest in this context. In confessing some apprehension at finding himself in close proximity to his Highland hosts, he adds that 'a young Highlander is always somewhat suspicious as to scorbutic symptoms;' thus revealing both that scurvy was to be expected in the Highlanders and his belief that it was contagious. Boswell also makes the interesting comment that on an island as remote as Raasay 'there is a great plenty of potatoes'. (For further discussion on scurvy see Chapter 4 under 'Vegetables and Fruit'.)

Looking next at vitamin A and recalling that it is found both in fatty, oily foods and in green and coloured vegetables, we find its score to be low in our chosen menu, moderate amounts only being supplied by dairy products and kail. In attempting to estimate the probable intake of vitamin D, we are of course faced with an imponderable—the degree of exposure to sunlight: apart from this, the content is certainly low. What is worthy of note, however, is that both of these vitamins—vital factors for growth—can be stored in the body, which means that even an occasional feast (of liver perhaps, or a fatty fish like herring, or even eggs) could well have provided a useful reservoir to see the people through their hard times.

There does certainly seem to have been plenty of salmon, a rich source of vitamins A and D. Perhaps, in some places, there may have been so much that even our undemanding ancestors could tire of it, although some writers have complained that this is a fiction originating with 'the overcredulous Burt'. That gentleman's well-known story on this point may nevertheless bear re-telling.

> The meanest Servants, who are not at Board-wages, will not make a Meal upon Salmon if they can get any Thing else to eat. I have been told it here, as a very good Jest, that a Highland Gentleman, who went to London by Sea, soon after his Landing passed a Tavern where the Larder appeared to the Street, and operated so strongly upon his Appetite that he went in—that there were among other Things a Rump of Beef and some Salmon: of the Beef he ordered a Steak for himself, 'but,' says he, 'let Duncan have some Salmon.' To be short, the Cook who attended him humoured the Jest, and the Master's eating was eight Pence, and Duncan's came to almost as many Shillings.[5]

It seems clear that, at least when times were good, the diet of the Scots rural workers was in most respects a highly nourishing one, and here it might be as well to leave it. It should be added, however, that the nineteenth century did bring some important changes, at least in some areas. First, meat foods—venison, mutton, poultry, hares, rabbits—became more widely available. Also, improvements in the realm of cottage gardening led to an increase in the variety of produce, and not least in the vitamin C-rich fruits (black and red currants and gooseberries) as well as a larger selection of vegetables. From this time onwards, particularly after sugar came into more common use, what amounted to a mini-revolution in the culinary arts began to take place. Jams, jellies and marmalades were produced everywhere, in addition to the wide selection of baked items and puddings for which the Scots would eventually become famous.

Of the latter part of the century Henry Graham in *The Social Life of Scotland* says:

> Other things had changed in the social condition of the people, and had changed mostly for the better. The fare was no longer restricted to the monotonous oat and barley bread in all its forms. In the kailyard, there was no longer a meagre supply of vegetables, chiefly cabbage and greens; but turnips, carrots, potatoes and many others in which they took pride and loved to cultivate, along with the currant and gooseberry bushes, and roses, and beloved peppermint. The use of these had, it was said, a markedly favourable effect upon the health of the peasantry.[6]

And later, in the *Appendix to the General Report of Scotland*, 1814, we find cottage gardeners being advised that 'the fittest articles of produce are summer cabbage, winter kail, a few early potatoes, turnips, beans, leeks and onions.'[7] They are urged, too, to plant early potatoes for use in summer when oatmeal would be at its dearest, and so that winter greens could then be planted in the limited space available.

How were the more opulent classes faring as the far-reaching changes of the eighteenth century were taking place? Due to the burgeoning of trade and consequent greater availability of cash, the whole social scene was undergoing transformation: the frugal, unpretentious manner of life of country society was gradually disappearing, largely through the influence of wider education and travel. More imposing, and comfortable, houses were being built; manners were becoming more polished; inevitably the food, too, began to become more sophisticated. Extensive gardens and orchards for fruit, flowers and vegetables were at the same time being laid out, thus paving the way for Scotland's future market gardening renown.

The profligate hospitality of the era is summed up thus by Graham:

> The spirit of those old days was eminently hospitable, and exuberantly hearty. . . . Neighbours were wont to come, without sending word, on horseback; and in the effusiveness of hospitality there was shown a 'pressing' of guests to stay, which it was a meanness to omit and offence to resist. The bashful ate till full to repletion; the amiable and obsequious fed in meek compliance; the stalwart only dared to refuse, and the prudent saved themselves by keeping something always on their plate. . . . Then, as always, were the inevitable dishes—broth, beef and hens.[8]

Clearly belonging to this hospitable era is the ample meal

produced at night—and impromptu—for Captain Brown by
Dandie Dinmont's gudewife, in Scott's *Guy Mannering*:

> Two fowls, a huge piece of cold beef-ham, eggs, butter, cakes, and
> barley-meal bannocks in plenty . . . diluted with home-brewed ale of
> excellent quality, and a case-bottle of brandy.[9]

Even with the help of the deep-freeze, few modern housewives
could hope to rise to such heights.

In order to observe the gradual change from plain to more
sophisticated eating which came about as the eighteenth century
wore on, it is interesting to note some of the menus quoted by
Graham as typical of the establishment of a 'modest laird' of the
era, looking first at the early part of the century and then towards
the end.[10]

Early 18th century

5—6 a.m.	The laird rose and took his 'morning'—a glass of whisky or brandy
8 a.m. *Breakfast*	'Skink' [water gruel] Collops or mutton with ale Barley or oatmeal bannocks [Wheaten bread on special occasions only]
12 noon—1 p.m. *Dinner*	'Monotonous fare' of broth of beef or mutton made with barley groats Fresh meat summer and autumn only; otherwise salt meat and 'kain hens' [given in rent by tenants] Game on special days *Note*: No vegetables served except kail, or 'neeps' in broth. No sweets or puddings. To drink—ale, sack or claret.
'4 Hours'	Some refreshment for all—ale and wine for ladies; wheaten bread, as a delicacy, if guests present [Tea, at first violently opposed as a 'vile drug' and capable of producing 'tremblings and shakings of the head and hands, loss of appetite, vapours and other nervous diseases', gradually gained in popularity and by mid-century was firmly entrenched]
7—8 p.m. *Supper*	Another substantial meal, more or less identical with dinner—broth, fresh or salt meat and hens Ale, sack or claret

It need scarcely be pointed out that variety was somewhat lacking in this type of fare, as Graham makes abundantly clear when he writes:

> With pitiless monotony, day by day and month by month, families patiently subsisted until the cattle, having returned to pasture, were restored to health, and they could get fresh beef again. Besides this stale diet there were the 'kain hens', which formed part of the laird's rent from his tenants—food which became no less intolerably tiresome to the palate. . . . Vegetables were not served on table, potatoes and turnips being almost unattainable; and the 'neeps' or parsnips or greens were only used as ingredients in the kail. Sweets there were none: dessert was unknown.

Taken all in all, is it perhaps possible that the cottagers in some ways fared better?

But all this, too, was to change. Moving on to the end of the century, we find that the tastes of the rural gentry had become more delicate. Gone now, in great measure, was the habit of grossly over-spicing meat to disguise its extreme saltiness; gone too, as Graham puts it, 'the unfailing broth, salt meat and hens'. We begin indeed to see the first intimations of modern menu-planning, food no longer being served in one vast miscellaneous course, including roast and boiled meats side by side. Vegetables begin to be served along with meats, and puddings and desserts—common enough in Edinburgh society from the time of Mary Queen of Scots—make their belated appearance. As for the beverages, one cannot help feeling that at least they were sufficiently plentiful to wash down even the toughest of meat and to disguise the most unattractive of flavours. In the early nineteenth century, Sir Walter Scott, in his novel *Guy Mannering,* makes this very point, showing that these social advances were not confined to the lairds:

> The present store-farmers of the south of Scotland are a much more refined race than their fathers . . . without losing the rural simplicity of manners, they now cultivate arts unknown to the former generation, not only in the progressive improvement of their possessions, but in all the comforts of life. Their houses are more commodious . . . and the best of luxuries, the luxury of knowledge, has gained much ground. Deep drinking, formerly their greatest failing, is now fast losing ground, and, while the frankness of their extensive hospitality continues the same, it is, generally speaking, refined in its character, and restrained in its excesses.[11]

The largely self-supporting nature of gentlemen's establishments is made very evident in the *Memoirs of a Highland Lady*:

At this time in the Highlands we were so remote from markets we had to depend very much on our own produce for most of the necessaries of life. Our flocks and herds supplied us not only with the chief part of our food, but with fleeces to be wove into clothing, blanketing, and carpets, horn for spoons, leather to be dressed at home for various purposes, hair for the masons. We brewed our own beer, made our bread, made our candles; nothing was brought from afar but wine, groceries, and flour, wheat not ripening well so high above the sea. Yet we lived in luxury, game was so plentiful, red-deer, roe, hares, grouse, ptarmigan, and partridge; the river provided trout and salmon, the different lochs pike and char; the garden abounded in common fruit and common vegetables; cranberries and raspberries ran over the country, and the poultry-yard was ever well furnished. The regular routine of business, where so much was done at home, was really a perpetual amusement. I used to wonder when travellers asked my mother if she did not find her life dull.[12]

We now pass on to the kind of menu to which our 'modest Laird' and his household might have progressed by the closing years of the century, quoting again from Henry Graham:[13]

Sunday
Dinner	Cockyleekie soup	2 bottles claret
	Boiled beef and greens	2 bottles white wine
	Roast goose with potatoes	2 bottles strong ale
Supper	Mutton stewed with turnips	1 bottle claret
	Drawn eggs	1 bottle white wine
		1 bottle strong ale

Monday
Dinner	Pea soup	2 bottles claret
	Boiled turkey	2 bottles white wine
	Roast beef and greens	2 bottles strong ale
	Apple pie	
Supper	Mutton steaks, gravy potatoes	1 bottle claret
	Drawn eggs	1 bottle white wine
		1 bottle strong ale

It seems a little strange that in these excerpts no mention is made of breakfast, since Scotland was by this time becoming renowned for the excellence of this meal. Some travellers have left us mouth-watering descriptions, drawing particular attention to the new Scots delicacy, marmalade. A description by one James Bertram in his memoirs runs: 'A bitter-sweet but most delightful compound of orange skins and juices, called 'marmalade', which we never see in England.'

Dr Johnson, although not given to undue appreciation or praise of the general run of Scottish food, had some flattering things to say about the breakfasts.

> Not long after the dram may be expected the breakfast, a meal at which the Scots, whether of the Lowlands or mountains, must be confessed to excel us. The tea and coffee are accompanied not only with butter, but with honey, conserves, and marmalades. If an epicure could remove by a wish, in quest of sensual gratifications, wherever he had supped he would breakfast in Scotland.[14]

It should perhaps be recalled that the learned doctor had the good fortune to enjoy hospitality, apart from a few sojourns at inns of varying standards, in the houses of the great. Only once does he appear to have been offended—and surely not without cause—when his Hebridean hostess had the temerity to offer him some cold sheep's head for breakfast.

His companion James Boswell waxes most eloquent upon the breakfast provided in the Chief's residence on the island of Raasay. After an early morning drink of goat's whey, he partook of an excellent breakfast:

> as good chocolate as I ever tasted, tea, bread and butter, marmalade and jelly. There was no loaf-bread, but very good scones, or cakes of flour baked with butter . . . there were also barley-bannocks of this year's meal, and—what I cannot help disliking to have at breakfast—cheese. It is the custom all over the Highlands to have it; and it often smells very strong, and poisons to a certain degree the elegance of an Indian [exotic] breakfast.[15]

In view of the fact that magnificent breakfasts seem to have been the norm among the wealthier people of Scotland, it comes as something of a disappointment to find that this does not at all seem to have been true of her inns. To quote Graham again:

> In consequence of the small number of passengers on the roads in those days of bad travelling, the inns of Scotland were miserable in the extreme. . . . The Englishman, as he saw the servants without shoes or stockings, as he looked at the greasy tables without a cover, and saw the butter thick with cow-hairs, the coarse meal served without a knife and fork, so that he had to use his fingers or a clasp-knife, the one glass or tin handed round the company from mouth to mouth, his gorge rose.[16]

Nor do things seem to have improved much by the beginning of the next century. Dr John Macculloch, writing of a breakfast eaten at Taynuilt, in Argyll, before an ascent of Ben Cruachan in 1811, describes it thus: 'Musty bread, paste-like toast, cold herring, tepid tea and "damp and melancholy" sugar.'[17] Even less flattering is Dorothy Wordsworth's description of breakfast at Inveroran Inn, again in Argyll, in 1803: 'The butter not eatable, the barley-cakes fusty, the oat-bread so hard I could not chew it; and there were only four eggs in the house, which they had boiled as hard as stones.'[18] In contrast, Dr Johnson and Mr Boswell appeared to have fared reasonably well in at least some of the establishments in which they stayed; at an inn near Fort Augustus, for example, they were regaled on mutton chops, a broiled chicken, bacon and eggs, and a fricassee of moorfowl—surely no mean repast by any standards.

Looking again, however, at the gradually improving eating pattern in the houses of the country gentry, and in particular at the welcome change in winter from salted to fresh meat, we find that this quite clearly did not refer to all. Graham has some amusing anecdotes of those 'quaint-fashioned gentry who followed the olden ways'. To them the change to killing animals as required, even in winter so as to enjoy the luxury of fresh meat, would have seemed like wanton wastefulness. Salt meat they had always had, and salt meat they would continue to endure, if not to enjoy. Graham tells of a certain country gentleman

> who, with his docile household, methodically ate the animal from nose to tail, going down one side and up the other, till, to the relief of the family, the salt carcase was finished, only, however, to make way for another.[19]

Dean Ramsay tells a similar tale in his *Reminiscences of Scottish Life and Character*. The anecdote concerns a Scottish judge who gave a dinner party:

> When the covers were removed, the dinner was seen to consist of veal broth, a roast fillet of veal, veal cutlets, a florentine (an excellent old Scottish dish composed of veal), a calf's head, calf's foot jelly. The worthy judge could not help observing a surprise on the countenance of his guests, and perhaps a simper on some, so he broke out in explanation, 'Ou aye, it's a cauf. When we kill a beast, we just eat up ae side and doun the tither'.[20]

What, finally, of the nutritional value of the diet normally consumed by these rural lairds and their families? In the face of such a plethora of provisions it might seem superfluous even to comment: imbalance and even deficiency can, all the same, occur whenever awareness of nutritional values is lacking. It is at least possible, for example, that from time to time a deficiency of vitamin C may have occurred even among them, particularly in the earlier part of the century when vegetables were scarce. Again one is hampered by lack of exact knowledge of quantities consumed; most accounts nevertheless give a fairly clear impression that they were ample, not to say vast. While the intake of sweet and, to a lesser extent, starchy foods must surely have been much lower than that of most of us today, it is probable that that of fat was considerably higher. Certainly it is unlikely that anyone would have gone short of protein, calcium, iron or fat-soluble vitamins. Possibly the principal difference between their diet and that of the 'well-fed' Scots of today would be the fibre content: in the eighteenth century oatmeal and barley bannocks, supplying not only plenty of fibre but the important B group of vitamins as well, were common to lairds and tenants alike.

Ample as the fare in the houses of Scotland's lairds and smaller gentry may appear to us, it is when we turn to look at the food of her nobility that we meet with a degree of refinement and delicacy which may well take us wholly by surprise. And what is altogether most noteworthy is the fact that we do not, as might have been expected from the foregoing, have to wait until the end of the century to find it. One group of documents shedding unique light upon social life, and especially eating habits, are the Household Books of some of Scotland's stately homes. One such is the *Ochtertyre House Booke of Accomps*,[21] belonging to the baronial family of the Murrays of Ochtertyre, in Perthshire, who generously made it available for publication. It comprises a series of detailed menus for both gentry and servants, spanning the years 1737–9, and was written by one who was clearly a most meticulous household economist. It provides so much of rare interest that an apparent break in chronology may perhaps be forgiven.

And how much, apart from mere menus, filters through to us from those laboriously hand-written records of household expenses! Here indeed are all the fascinating details of early eighteenth-century life on a great Scottish estate. From the frequent entries for 'barm', for example, we learn that yeast baking was largely done at home, although in the latter part of the book there are recorded purchases of 'loves, rolls, biskits, bakes and nackits'. Home brewing—universal at the time—is evidenced by purchases of 'hoaps', and 'to the cooper for girding and repairing the brewhouse tubs'; while we also find numerous entries for a 'stoup of barm and corks 2 gross'. Of tea, the drink which would soon oust ale from Scots houses, there is mention only twice, in a reference to 'mending the tea-kettle'. Not surprisingly, considering its prime importance at the time, there is much about pickling of meat—in such items as 'brimston for the beefe', and 'lippies', 'pecks', and 'firlots' of salt. That the estate handyman was often occupied as butcher is shown by the many records of killings of livestock, as well as by the detail of his having been supplied with 'a sticking knife, a cliver and a slachter axe'. It is interesting to find that cheese appears on the gentry's menus scarcely at all—only five times in the entire book—but for the servants it is a common item; eggs, on the contrary, were bought on a vast scale, as many as 60 dozen in some of the months. Fish is well represented, too, and not simply locally-caught salmon and trout, but, thanks no doubt to the services of the cadgers, a large selection of both white fish and shellfish, and even occasionally a purchase of 'dulse and tangle'.

Noteworthy above all else, however, is the wide variety of vegetables figuring on the menus, in particular when one recalls the general dearth of these foods in that era. We find mention of broccoli, asparagus, artichokes, French beans, celery, spinach, mushrooms, and even salads of various types—some of which, it has to be confessed, would still have to be classed as minority tastes in present-day Scotland.

The pleasantries of local social exchange are evident in such snippets as the entry for June 1737: 'Received 33 wild-fowl from the hills, sent away 18 of them in compliments.' Gifts appear indeed to have been generally of food—shoulders of mutton, pieces of salmon, pigeons, trout, occasionally even a side of beef.

The menus themselves strike one most by their range and variety, especially in view of the grinding monotony we have been observing elsewhere. The standard, however, does tend to vary somewhat, possibly depending on the presence of 'company'; while the fact that some of the most elaborate meals are served on Sundays is unexpected, in that frugal fare was the general rule on that day among Presbyterian families.

The following are three menus from the book, each representing a different degree of grandeur:

Sunday 25 September 1737
    Dinner   Skink and tripe
                Beefe rost pieces
                Hams boyld

Tongues and lure
Hard fish and a plumb pudding
Calves head hasht and peas
Partridges with cellery
Turkeyes rost and larded
Geess rost
Pidgeons rost
Tarts and collard pige
Beefe for servants pieces

Supper   Veall rost joints
Pidgeons in a pye
Spinage and eggs and artichoaks
Puddings smoakt beefe and pickles
Foulls for broath

Saturday 29 January 1738
Dinner   Cockie leekie foulls in it
Pork boyld pieces
Hare collops and a pease pudding
Turkeyes rost
Mutton rost joints
Partridges stewd
Tarts and ane omlite
Mutton for servants and broath joints

Supper   Fish broyld
Cold turkey tarts hogs cheek and eggs
Smoak beefe and butter

Monday 16 January 1738
Dinner   Green keall
Foulls rost
Beefe for servants pieces

Supper   Collops
Mutton rost joints
Eggs and sallad magundey
Foulls for broath
Ducks in a pye

Certainly the ingredients of an excellent diet are to be found here, provided of course that choice was prudent. By and large, all the same, it is reasonable to suppose that some at least of those amply-nourished lords and ladies might well have been subject, even if shielded to some extent by the comparative absence of stress and strain in their lives, to those ills attendant upon over-nutrition which are causing concern in the affluent lifestyle of the present day.

4

THE SCOTS LARDER

What foods were on its shelves?

What were our ancestors' principal foods, from mediaeval times onward? Most people faced with this question will begin by quoting foods of animal origin—venison, mutton, haggis, herrings, black puddings and the like—and will then go on to mention barley and oatmeal. This is the wrong way round. Apart from dairy products, the supply of which varied according to the prevailing degree of prosperity, by far the major part of the rural diet consisted of various types of meal, produced by grinding not only oats and barley but also more unusual crops like pease (split peas) and beans. In looking, therefore, at the commoner items found in the Scots larder of bygone days, it seems fitting to consider cereals and dairy produce first, and meat and fish later. Fruits and vegetables never did figure prominently in the diet, but we shall finally take a look at those few which did.

CEREALS AND PULSES

Dr Samuel Johnson, in 1773, comments upon the absence of yeast bread in Scotland. 'Their native bread,' he observes, 'is made of oats or barley. Of oatmeal they spread very thin cakes, coarse and hard, to which unaccustomed palates are not easily reconciled.'[1] (Is it perhaps a little unkind to wonder whether he is thinking even more of unaccustomed teeth?) The learned doctor continues:

> The barley cakes are thicker and softer; I began to eat them without unwillingness; the blackness of their colour raises some dislike, but the taste is not disagreeable. In most houses there is wheat flour, with which we were sure to be treated, if we staid long enough to have it kneaded and baked. As neither yeast nor leaven is used among them their bread of every kind is unfermented. They make only cakes, and never mould a loaf.

The reason was that wheat flour was scarce and expensive, nor did most people have ovens in which to bake it. Instead they made bannocks on a simple iron girdle. That Dr Johnson was constantly being offered wheaten cakes is a pointer to the traditional hospitality of his hosts, for these were generally reserved for special occasions.

Dr Johnson was of course writing of the Highlands and Islands. Elsewhere the situation was not necessarily the same. Although grown from the time of the Cistercian farmer-monks in the fertile areas (notably the South-East, the North-East, and the Carse of Gowrie), wheat normally found its way to the tables of the higher classes, either via their own ovens or the town bake-ovens, thus inevitably becoming a prestige food. Wheat bread is mentioned in some mediaeval records—for example, in The Records of Elgin, 1234–1800,[2] under 'the prices of victuallis in the market . . . the loaf of good wheat bread to cost 4d', the year being 1556. And records of St Andrews University for the year 1597 show that masters and regents received an allowance of wheat bread each day, along with beef, mutton, fish, eggs and ale; while bursars and servants had oat bread instead of wheat.

Tracing the pattern of bread-eating through different areas and social classes, and noting especially its eventual fall in the social scale, makes an interesting study (see Chapter 5). Account must be taken, however, of the earlier cereals over which wheat gradually took precedence in Scotland. These were barley (or bere) and oats.

Although to most people the cereal most readily associated with Scotland was oats, prior to the eighteenth century at least barley was a popular food, being used not only for making bannocks and porridge but also in the brewing of ale and distilling of whisky. Records do show, all the same, that the bulk of the barley crop was in fact used for food. In the Highlands and among the poorer folk, barley porridge and bannocks continued as basic foods until well into the nineteenth century. In the Orkney Islands and Caithness bere-bannocks are still eaten, although in a more sophisticated form.

It should not be forgotten that a considerable proportion of the barley used would have been incorporated in broth, always a popular dish in the Highlands especially. Somewhat surprisingly, we find that this was an item which found great favour with Samuel Johnson. Boswell writes:

> At dinner Dr Johnson ate several platefuls of Scotch broth with pease in them, and was very fond of the dish. I said, 'you never ate it before, sir.' 'No, sir, but I don't care how soon I eat it again.'[3]

One wonders how much of an appetite he could possibly have had after several platefuls of such filling food.

Gradually, from the eighteenth century onwards, oatmeal began to assume its place as Scotland's favourite cereal food. Despite the fact that barley has now reappeared as a 'health food', the truth is that in nearly every nutritional aspect oatmeal is superior, containing one and a half times as much protein (significant in view of the dearth of animal foods in the diet of those days), as well as substantially more iron, calcium and vitamin B_1.

Writing from Inverness in the early part of the eighteenth century, Captain Burt was not slow to observe an undue dependence upon oatmeal:

> By the small Proportion the arable Lands hereabout bear to the rocky Grounds and barrren Heaths, there is hardly a Product of Grain sufficient to supply the Inhabitants, let the Year be ever so favourable; and therefore, any ill Accident that happens to their Growth, or Harvest, produces a melancholy Effect. I have known, in such a Circumstance, the Town being in Consternation for Want of Oatmeal, when Shipping has been retarded, and none to be procured for Love nor Money. There are but few in this Town that eat Wheat-bread, besides the English and those that belong to them, and some of the principal Inhabitants, but not their Servants.[4]

Ideally suited as it was to the cottage with only the most basic of cooking equipment (normally a solid iron plate or girdle and an iron kail-pot, both of which hung over the open fire by a swey or chain), oatmeal came in time to be used for a wide variety of regional dishes. Most commonly it became either thin oatcakes or thicker bannocks, or else porridge, brose, or sowens. This last was made by soaking the mealy husk of ground oats in a tub of water for several days until fermentation had begun; then sieving and finally boiling the resultant mixture with water and salt to produce a kind of thin porridge which was believed (probably with good reason) to be particularly suitable for invalids.

The *Statistical Account* for Bendothy, in Perthshire, comments:

> The common people live on oatmeal pottage twice a-day. It is the most wholesome and palatable of all their food, being purely vegetable; notwithstanding the reflection in Johnson's Dictionary, that 'oats are eaten by horses in England, and in Scotland by men.' Such food makes men strong like horses, and purges the brain of pedantry.[5]

The vital part played by oats in Scotland is summed up comprehensively by David Kerr Cameron in his fascinating history of the

Scottish farmtouns which had their heyday from about the 1880s onwards.

> Oatmeal was the great sustainer: there was never a time in Scotland's long history when a little meal in your poke was not better than coin in your pouch. It was more than a food; it was a currency that in its time was a unit of rent; the stipends of ministers; the fees of schoolmasters; and payment for hardy Highland postmen. Gamekeepers sent into the hills for something to fill the chief's pot took oatmeal in their pockets—their only provision on an expedition that might stretch over several nights in the open before they brought home the venison. Like the laird's firlot or two of barley or oats to the tradesmen, oatmeal honourably settled debt and was welcome as dowries. About the farmtouns it was both a scourge and the very substance of life itself. And as a part of his perquisites, it was an important part of the ploughman's fee.
>
> The men of the farmtouns, in fact, lived on an infinity of [oatmeal] brose: brose when they fell out of their beds in the morning, kail brose for their 'denner'—the midday meal—and oatmeal brose again for their supper, when they had stabled their horses for the night. . . . The standard dish of the bothymen, and one just right for the haste of a farmtoun morning, was oatmeal mixed with boiling water, with salt and pepper added, and taken with cream or milk. You could, if you had a mind to, sugar it, lace it with treacle, instead of the milk even have stout or porter. It wasn't haute cuisine, yet generations of farmtoun men marched on it to the very endrigs of life itself and were seemingly none the worse for it, except for the occasional outbreak of the euphemistically-named Scotch fiddle, a skin eruption brought on it was thought by the unrelieved diet of oatmeal.[6]

Rye, although grown in Scotland from early times, does not seem ever to have been eaten to the same extent as in other countries of Northern Europe, where its use has continued up to the present day. Indeed, it is interesting to speculate whether consumption here may not have reached a higher level in our present era of slimming and rye crispbreads.

Two rather more unlikely bread-crops were pease and beans, the ground meal of which was mixed with barley to make a kind of flour. Peasemeal, used again for the making of the ever-popular brose, was in demand until the Second World War, but is difficult to come by today.

Peas and beans, like all pulses, are rich in protein, one ounce of each giving approximately as much of this vital bodybuilding nutrient as one egg, and in addition they supply iron and some vitamins of the B group; so their contribution to the diet in days gone by was far from negligible.

Clearly then our rural forefathers had much cause to be grateful for their native-grown cereals and pulse foods, which were indeed excellent complements to each other. It is, however, to the partnership of cereal foods with dairy products that the high quality of the country people's diet must chiefly be ascribed.

MILK, BUTTER AND CHEESE

Through the centuries, ever since the first pastoral peoples reached our shores, milk and its products have formed a vital part of our country's food.

Many writings make it clear that milk was the mainstay of the diet in early times, and not simply cows' milk, but also that of goats and sheep. In 1773 Dr Johnson saw both sheep and goats being milked in Skye. Goats must in fact have been particularly numerous in Scotland, to judge by the number of times the Gaelic word 'gabhar' appears in the names of our hills; large herds of wild goats do still frequent many of our mountainous areas. Dr Johnson, in describing his host in Glenmoriston, writes: 'His life seemed to be merely pastoral, except that he differed from some of the ancient Nomades in having a settled dwelling. His wealth consists of a hundred sheep, as many goats, twelve milk-cows, and 28 beeves ready for the drover.'[7] Goats' milk was used principally for cheesemaking, but was also drunk as such or in the form of goat-whey; the *Statistical Account* reports that 'consumptives' were often sent to Dunkeld for the summer months to drink this beverage. Again Dr Johnson comments: 'The milk of goats is much thinner than that of cows, and that of sheep is much thicker. Sheep's milk is never eaten before it is boiled; as it is thick, it must be very liberal of curd, and the people of St Kilda form it into small cheeses.'

In the farming communities of the pre-enclosure days, the right to graze a cow was of prime importance, milk being vital in keeping hunger at bay. At those times when milk was virtually the only available food, it was customary to beat it to a froth with a special stick in order to increase its bulk, a practice which obviously added nothing to its nutritional value.

Inevitably a wide range of regional milk dishes evolved around the country, incorporating not only milk itself but also cream, buttermilk, whey and curds. Milk was either drunk on its own or used with porridge and brose, or at times added to broths; cereal puddings did not become popular till the nineteenth century. Dr Johnson, writing of the Hebrides, observes:

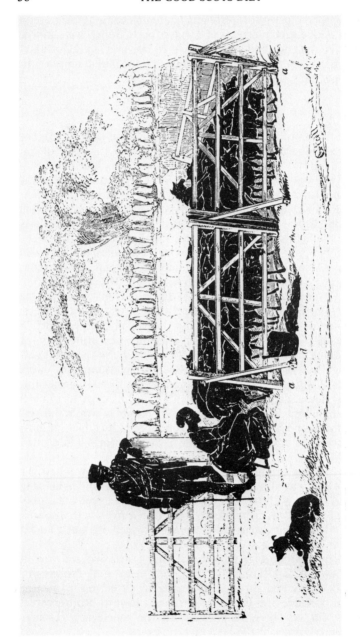

1   Milking Ewes. From H Stephens, *The Book of the Farm*, 2nd edn II (1985), 221. *Source* National Museum of Antiquities of Scotland C6679.

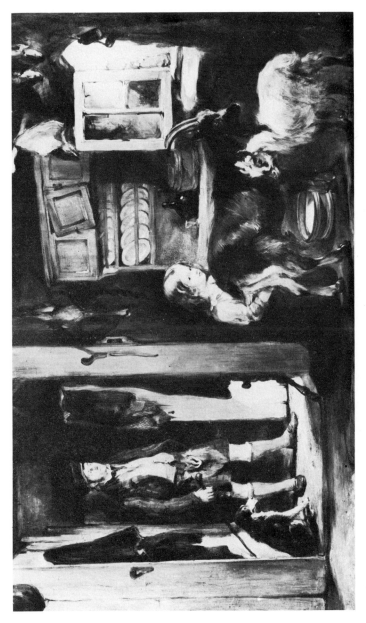

2　Goatherd's cottage, painted by D Simpson, 1832. *Source* National Galleries of Scotland, Edinburgh, C4167.

A dinner in the Western Islands differs very little from a dinner in England, except that in the place of tarts, there are always set preparations of milk. This part of their diet will stand some improvement. Though they have milk and eggs, and sugar, few of them know how to compound them into a custard.

It would indeed seem a natural thing to combine milk and eggs into custards, and certainly it looks as if these were known in other parts of Scotland, since they are mentioned more than once in descriptions of the ancient Beltane customs, in the *Statistical Account*:

> Upon the first of May, which is called Beltan, or Baltein Day, all the boys in a township or hamlet, meet in the moors. . . . They kindle a fire, and dress a repast of milk and eggs in the consistence of a custard. They knead a cake of oatmeal, which is toasted at the embers against a stone. After the custard is eaten up, they divide the cake into so many portions, as similar as possible to one another in size and shape. Every one, blindfold, draws out a portion.[8]

Butter and various types of cheese have been made in Scotland from very early times. Not surprisingly , we find that butter caused our ancestors a great deal of bother through its being so perishable. Much ingenuity was required, and used, in attempting to overcome this difficulty; for example, the butter might be placed in a wooden container or wrapped in bark, and then immersed in a well or a bog. This was of course unsalted butter, salt being a scarce commodity: but later, salted butter which would keep fresh for considerably longer was sold in the towns.

What surprises us more today is the fact that, at least until the nineteenth century, barley bannocks and oatcakes were eaten dry, butter being reserved mainly for cooking purposes. Dry oatcakes at each meal would seem something less than alluring to most of us nowadays; when we consider, however, that making butter by the old hand-churning method took several hours, and that four gallons of cream produced only about 6 lb of butter, we can more easily understand—a salutary reminder to those who feel they are over-worked houswewives today.

In his booklet *Traditional Elements in the Diet of the Northern Isles of Scotland,* Alexander Fenton sheds interesting light on the practices associated with butter in these islands.

> Up to the nineteenth century the farmers' rents were paid partly in butter—the Orcadians made a distinction between 'meat' and 'grease' butter. Meat butter was the best quality, and was kept for home

consumption. The poorer quality grease butter was used to pay the rent. This was exported by the landlords, and was often used by lowland farmers for mixing with tar to smear their sheep.[9]

Corroboration of this last point comes from a manuscript study of the life and times of Mary Stewart (1767–1837),[10] a native of Glen Tarken, in Perthshire, written by her great-grandson in conjunction with Mrs N Watt of Comrie:

> Butter, on the farms, was used for cooking, but was not otherwise usually eaten; for the most part it was mixed with Archangel tar and smeared on sheep; the butter and the natural oil in the fleece gave resistance to wet, and the tar had an antiseptic quality.

Predictably, though, the scarcity of fat for cooking meant that such items as pastries and pies became luxury items: vegetable oils were not used at the time.

Several of the more fastidious early travellers in Scotland were repelled by the butter. One can sympathise with their complaint that it was invariably full of cows' hairs.

It is interesting to speculate upon the fat consumption of our rural ancestors. Their only really regular sources appear to have

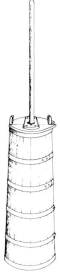

3   Plunge churn for making butter: in the National Museum. Drawn by C Hendry. *Source* National Museum of Antiquities of Scotland, C6792.

been butter and milk, along with occasional or small amounts of cheese. Fat intakes must therefore have been considerably lower than ours today: even with occasional additions like the fat from salmon, herrings, meat and eggs, the total must have been a modest one. Not so with the landlord classes, who must surely have faced a mini-mountain of dairy produce offered by their tenants in rent, as well as their daily fare of 'salt meat and kain hens', and who might well have had a fat intake exceeding that of even the most amply fed today.

Man has always, it seems, found ways of preserving milk. Primitive pastoral peoples still fill animal-skin bags with milk— from camels, ewes or goats—and hang them up until the milk is coagulated by bacterial action in the heat of the sun. Similar methods were doubtless employed in Scotland long ago. An early practice in Shetland, for example, was the making of a kind of cream cheese, known as 'hung milk', by filling a linen bag with milk and then leaving it until the whey had dripped away.

Normally, of course, the enzyme rennin from the stomach of a young animal is required to form the curd. The Scots of past centuries used a variety of stomachs—mainly those of lambs and pigs, but also of hares and deer—as well as an interesting selection of substances to add flavour and 'break the curd': examples are mustard, caraway seed and the ubiquitous oatmeal. Naturally, therefore, a wide selection of cheeses came to be produced, these tending on the whole to be soft cheese and crowdie in the Highlands, and the harder types—in which the whey was drained off— in the South. The by-product, whey, was in addition an important food for livestock. Native ingenuity, in some cases, overcame the problem posed by scarcity of salt, as when the St Kildan women used ashes of sea-weed in making their cheeses of ewes' milk.

That a good deal of the cheese eaten by rural folk in the eighteenth century was made from skimmed milk seems not unlikely: an entry in the *Statistical Account* (Perthshire) notes that 'there is a good deal of butter and cheese made; but the cheese is less valuable than it would be, by lacking the substance of the butter.'[11] A valuable food, nevertheless, it undoubtedly was, whether made from whole milk or not; providing weight for weight approximately as much protein as meat; along with much calcium and some vitamins. What is difficult to establish from this distance is the actual extent to which cheese was included in the ordinary folk's diet; in the typical menus of the day it is not very often quoted. Probably cottars were glad to sell their kebbocks of cheese to raise badly-needed cash; let us hope, all the same, that they were able to retain sufficient of this excellent food to help with the feeding of their families.

It would be difficult to leave the subject of dairy foods without a brief backward look at one very special feature of Scottish rural life which has now vanished, but which in some cases lasted up to the present century—the summer shielings, called in Gaeilic *airidhean*. The celebrated eighteenth-century traveller Thomas Pennant makes mention of these when writing of Glen Tilt, in Perthshire:

> Ascend a steep hill, on the top of which we refreshed ourselves with some goat's whey, at a SHEELIN, or, as it is sometimes called, ARRIE or BOTHAY, a dairy house, where the Highland shepherds, or graziers, live during summer with their herds and flocks, and during that season make butter and cheese. Their whole furniture consists of a few horn spoons, their milking utensils, a couch formed of sods to lie on, and a rug to cover them. Their food oatcakes, butter or cheese, and often the coagulated blood of their cattle spread on their bannocks. They drink milk, whey, and sometimes by way of indulgence, whisky.[12]

A less primitive way of living, however, was general in later times; what amounted to a kind of mass 'flitting' took place annually, when all the inhabitants of a small township or village— men, women and children—would load on to their carts (or backs) bedding, provisions, tools, dairy utensils and spinning equipment, and would depart with their livestock for the simple dwellings up in the hills, where the women and children were to spend the summer. On the first good day of early summer they would be off, with excitement running high and everyone in good spirits. (The present writer may be forgiven a possibly over-romanticised view due to the half-remembered tales of a Highland grandmother, but it is easy to think somewhat wistfully of the wholesome simplicity of a vanished way of life, and indeed to wonder whether modern luxury holidays ever generated half as much joyful enthusiasm.)

Arrived at the huts, the men would set about carrying out any necessary repairs, and would then partake of a simple meal, pausing to pray God's blessing on the summer's work before departing for the deserted township; leaving behind women and young folk to herd the cattle on the upland pastures, make the cheese and butter, and collect herbs and roots for dyeing. Over the ensuing months fare would be of the simplest, principally milk and whey and oatmeal, and perhaps some wild fruits, supplemented possibly by occasional catches of game. Down in the glens the men-folk would live equally simply, tending their crops in the welcome

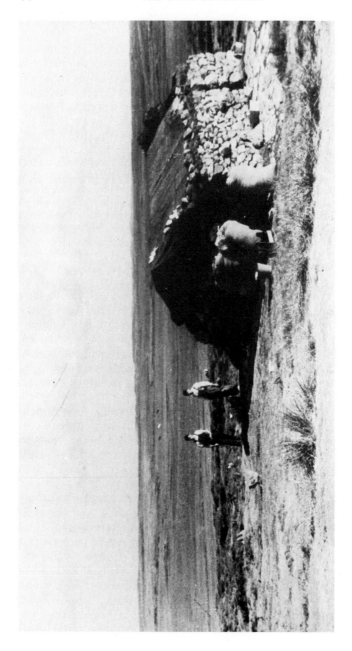

4   'Typical Moorland Shielding, Lewis'. Photograph A M Macdonald, ARPS Stornoway. 45/5/14. By kind permission of Rachel M Macdonald.

absence of wandering cattle-beasts; cleaning and re-thatching the houses (the old thatch being used as fertiliser), ready for the day when the whole operation would take place in reverse and the clean, re-furbished houses would again be filled with the bustle of an active, lively community.

FOWLS AND THEIR EGGS

Hens and geese were always kept in agricultural Scotland, often inhabiting the houses along with their owners, and were frequently included in rents paid in kind. Probably it was not often that they actually graced the tables of the cottars; the lairds and their families, on the other hand, must surely at times have been heartily sick of the taste of cockaleekie.

As with cheese, eggs are seldom quoted in the menus of the rural workers, and it is probably correct therefore to regard them, also, as occasional foods. It is known that they were often sold to travelling hawkers, known as 'egglers', who carried them to town markets in creels on their backs. In many places, particularly of course in islands and around the coast, the eggs of wild birds were commonly eaten: the practice of eating peewits' (lapwings) eggs is not uncommon even yet in some Highland areas; but much more generally it was the eggs of sea-birds—of gulls, guillemots and fulmars especially—which added a most nutritious supplement to the ordinary diet of the people. An outstanding exception is provided by St Kilda—admittedly representing a unique way of life—where, far from being merely a supplement, they provided a vital part of the basic diet. The economy of the island was indeed based largely upon sea-birds, notably puffins and fulmars—their flesh, their eggs, their oil and their feathers—the last two of which the St Kildans even managed to export.

Martin Martin in his account of a visit to St Kilda (c. 1695) makes intriguing mention of the vast numbers of sea-birds' eggs habitually consumed by the inhabitants of that island.

> We had the curiosity after three weeks' residence to make a calcule of the number of eggs bestowed upon those in our boat, and the Stewart's birlin, or galley; the whole amounted to sixteen thousand eggs; and without all doubt the inhabitants, who were treble our number, consumed many more eggs and fowls than we could.[13]

Tom Steel, in *The Life and Death of St Kilda*, gives a vivid description of the fulmar catch on the island, that highly dangerous undertaking which provided the people with **hair-raising** adventures, but also with vital food:

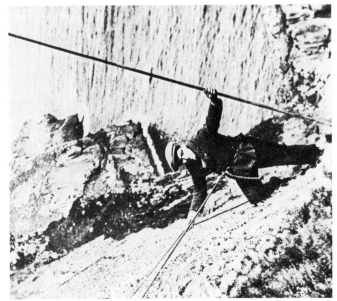

6 Fowling with rope and fowling rod on the St Kilda cliffs. Photograph A M Macdonald, ARPS, Stornoway. C1014. By kind permission of Rachel M Macdonald.

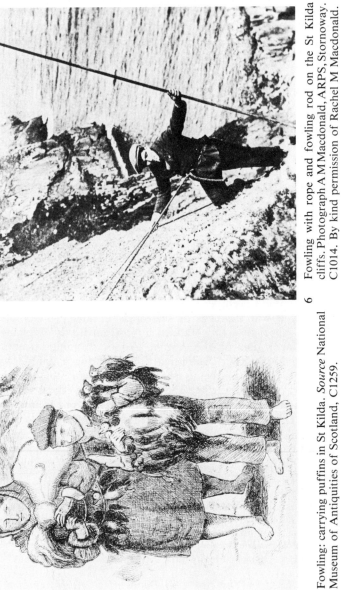

5 Fowling: carrying puffins in St Kilda. *Source* National Museum of Antiquities of Scotland, C1259.

Every evening during the harvest, the fulmars were divided equally among the islanders, and after the division, each share was carried back to its respective home where men, women and children would sit up often all night plucking the birds and preparing those that they wanted preserved for winter consumption. The feathers were carefully put aside for sale to the factor ; the vile-smelling oil, of which each bird yielded normally half a pint, was squeezed out and put into canisters, also for export; and the bird was then split lengthways down the back, the viscera removed and put upon the refuse heap to be used as manure at a later date, and if the islanders did not want to eat the flesh of the bird in the immediate future, the body was filled with salt. Thus prepared, thousands of birds were packed in barrels, like herring, for the winter.[14]

A magnificent example of skill, initiative and thrift.

We noted in an earlier chapter that the two nutrients likely to be deficient in the cereal-based rural diet were the important vitamins A and D. Eggs, which are good sources of these, would thus serve to make good the deficiencies.

The eating of various seabirds has clearly been a common practice in many parts of Scotland for centuries. In Orkney, for example, the flesh of the guillemot was considered a delicacy; young cormorants, too, were eaten after first being buried for twenty-four hours to tenderise them; in St Kilda, as we have just noted, fulmars and puffins were the important foods.

In the East Lothian area, gannets caught on the Bass Rock seem to have been highly prized as food, and the literature throws interesting light on this subject. A wildfowler known as The Climber of the Bass was for long employed to capture gannets on the cliffs, one old record giving his haul for a particular year as 1,118 birds. These sold for £79. 3s. 10d, his own salary being £11. 12s. 2d., not a particularly generous recompense for an occupation which, on the notoriously dangerous cliffs, is said to have killed at least one climber a year. John Taylor, a traveller to Scotland in 1618, ate solan goose (gannet) from the Bass Rock. He commented:

> It is very good flesh, but it is eaten in the forme wee eate oysters, standing at a side-board, a little before dinner, unsanctified without grace: and after it is eaten, it must be well liquoured with two or three good rowses of sherrie or Canarie sacke.[15]

One feels that might certainly have helped. He noted that the owner of the Bass made a profit in the region of two hundred pounds a year from his solan geese, surely no mean reward for those times.

The gannet, indeed, was regarded as a delicacy fit for even a royal table; nevertheless, King Charles II is quoted as remarking that there were two things he disliked in Scotland—the solan goose and the Solemn League and Covenant. A piece of roast gannet was considered a good appetiser; it is said, however, that a farmer attending a public dinner claimed to have eaten a whole gannet before leaving home, but found his appetite not a whit the keener for it.

Game-birds must regularly have graced the tables of the gentry, but would rarely be tasted by the ordinary folk. Dr Johnson (who, it must be remembered, was generally fortunate enough to be entertained by the gentry on his travels) made this observation on his Highland tour:

> At the tables where a stranger is received, neither plenty nor delicacy is wanting. A tract of land so thinly inhabited, must have much wild-fowl, and I scarce remember to have seen a dinner without them. The moorgame is everywhere to be had.[16]

FISH

Fish has always formed an important part of the Scots diet although, predictably, consumption varied a good deal according to location and availability.

Sea-fish—mainly haddock, cod and plaice—were prominent in the diet in coastal areas and indeed for some distance inland (possibly up to something in the order of 20 miles, depending on the range of those colourful characters who were so much part of the traditional scene, the Scots fishwives). Clearly the East Coast towns and villages were always well and cheaply served as regards fish; and where catches were too large for immediate consumption the excess was preserved for later use or for trading purposes by splitting, salting and drying the fish on shingly beaches. Dr Johnson must have encountered this, as his friend Boswell records:

> I bought some speldings, fish (generally whitings) salted and dried in a particular manner, being dipped in the sea and dried in the sun, and eaten by the Scots by way of a relish. He had never seen them, though they are sold in London. I insisted on *scottifying* his palate, but he was very reluctant. With difficulty I prevailed with him to let a bit of one of them lie in his mouth. He did not like it.[17]

In the Northern Isles and the Hebrides, too, fish played a vital part in filling the hungry gap between one harvest and the next.

These were principally coal-fish, known as sillocks, caught from the rocks with circular nets, or even at times with blankets, the people eating their flesh and using the oil from their livers as fuel for their lamps. It is at least possible that some of this valuable oil may have been wasted—a sad thought, in that such fish oils are a rich source of vitamin D, the very vitamin which could have prevented the cruel deformities suffered by thousands of children in the city slums.

It can readily be imagined that an easily accessible source of food such as the commoner shellfish round Highland and island shores must often have kept the common folk alive in days of over-population and under-nutrition.

Osgood Mackenzie of Gairloch writes:

> One has only to look at the sites of the shielings even some miles from the sea, where great heaps of shells tell their tale. Shell-fish boiled in milk was a great stand-by in those days. I sometimes wonder that they did not carry the milk down-hill to the coast, rather than carry the shell-fish up to the hills.

He tells, too, of 'the finest and strongest family of young men ever known at Poolewe', reared largely upon *maorach a'chladaich* (shell-fish of the shore), in this case limpets and white whelks.[18]

Fresh fish, particularly salmon and trout, must certainly have made a significant contribution to the diet in many inland areas: that the folk could even become tired of it sounds strangely in the ears of those of us for whom, today, it is a rare luxury. In his classic work *The Scottish Gael,* James Logan comments: 'In Aberdeenshire the servants, during the summer, had so much salmon that they refused to eat of it oftener than twice a week.'[19]

But on the West Coast at least the fish which added most to the frugal diet of the common people was unquestionably the herring. Commercial fisheries involving the herring go back relatively far: in the reign of Charles II a Society of Herring Fishers was established on the Clyde, Greenock becoming a key centre of the industry. Loch Fyne, too, was early known for its fat herrings, popularly known as Glasgow Magistrates, although at least one early traveller considered these under-commercialised. Thomas Newte, after his visit in 1785, wrote: 'Loch Fine, properly an arm of the sea, produces herrings in great abundance, but it seems the fisheries are not carried on to that extent they would admit of'.[20]

Because of the herrings' well-known (and inconvenient) habit of arriving periodically in great shoals, it is easy to understand how some technology for preserving surpluses came to be devised, and

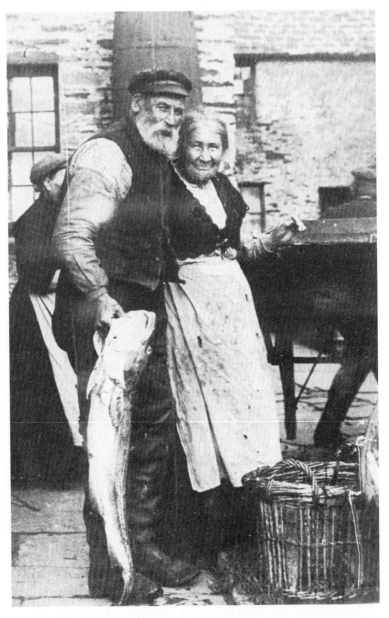

7   Fisher folk in Stromness, c.1900. Photograph G Ellison.

how this led eventually not only to each cottage having its own barrel of salt herrings as a bulwark against want, but also to the emergence of that succulent item so beloved of gourmets everywhere, the Scots kipper. It is of interest, however, that in earlier times the term 'kipper' frequently refers to salmon rather than herring. As has been pointed out in a previous chapter, the traditional cereal-based diet being short of vitamins A and D meant that herrings, richly endowed with these, could provide an excellent supplement. Alexander Fenton in *Scottish Country Life*[21] describes the delights of a meal of herrings and potatoes when cooked in the traditional Shetland manner—in a kail-pot over the open fire, with the herrings laid over the potatoes. Nutritionally, too, this is a meal which could scarcely be bettered.

The *Ochtertyre House Booke of Accomps* (1737–9)[22] sheds interesting light on the availability of fish in Scotland's great houses of the time. There seems indeed, judging by the recorded menus, to have been a fairly constant supply, doubtless through the useful offices of the cadgers. For example, we find 'harring' on the servants' menus in the first three months of the year and in July and August, as well as many other fish, including haddock, cod, sparlings, sole, whiting, skate, flounders, turbot, mackerel and dabs. Shell-fish such as oysters, mussels, lobsters and crabs (partons) also figure on the menus, while an intriguing entry appearing from time to time is 'a pennyworth of dulse and tangle'. 'It must have proved a good half hour's bargaining with the cadger,' observes the writer of the Introduction to the book, 'when my lady got 34 hadoes, a code, a string of whitens, and four partons for 1s. 7½d.'.

Seals and occasionally even whales were killed, for their oil as well as their flesh. In certain areas, too, both shellfish and sand-eels were undoubtedly used as food; yet more than one writer has made reference to the Scots' dislike of fish without scales, and particularly of eels. Some have claimed that both this and the traditional aversion to pork can be ascribed to the fact that the Scots following the Reformation were attempting adherence to Judaic law. 'The Scots have very recently divested themselves of many prejudices against certain fish', claims James Logan in *The Scottish Gael*, 'and those without scales are still disliked.'[23]

While it is clear that fish of various kinds must have figured fairly prominently in the traditional diet, what may not be so obvious is the scale on which fishing was carried on in some places. Thomas Pennant in his *Tour in Scotland*[24] notes of the city of Perth in 1772:

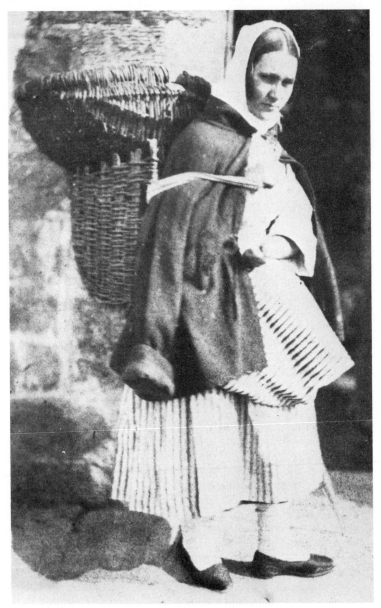

8   Fishwife with creel, Newhaven 18. Photograph D O Hill and R
Adamson. *Source* National Galleries of Scotland, Edinburgh.

It exports annually one hundred and fifty thousand pounds worth of linen, ten thousand of wheat and barley, and about the same in cured salmon. That fish is taken there in vast abundance; three thousand have been caught in one morning, weighing, one with another, sixteen pounds; the whole capture, forty-eight thousand pounds. Lough Tay abounds with Pike, Perch, Eels, Salmon and Trout; of the last, some have been taken that weighed above thirty pounds. Of these species, the Highlanders abhor eels, fancying, from the form, that they are too nearly related to serpents.

And of the fishing trade at Aberdeen:

The salmon fisheries on the Dee and the Don, are a good branch of trade; and in some years, one hundred and sixty-seven thousand pounds of fish have been sent pickled to London, and about nine hundred and thirty barrels of salted fish exported to France, Italy, etc.

We have already seen, on more than one occasion, that Captain Burt in his letters from the Highlands written in the early eighteenth century does little to endear himself to any Highlander, owing to his frequently critical and seemingly unsympathetic attitudes. Just for once, however, we may allow him to have the last word, on the subject of fish in Scotland. He writes:

This brings to Remembrance a Story I have heard of a Foreigner, who being duly arrived in this Country, at a public House desired something to eat. A Fowl was proposed, and accepted; but when it was dressed and brought to Table, the Stranger showed a great Dislike to it, which the Landlord perceiving, brought him a piece of fresh Salmon, and said 'Sir, I observe you do not like this Fowl; pray what do you think of this?' 'Think,' says the Stranger, 'Why, I think it is a very fine Salmon, and no Wonder, for that is of God Almighty's Feeding; if it had been by you, I suppose it would have been as lean as this poor Fowl, which I desire you will take away.[25]

MEAT AND ITS PRODUCTS

It would be interesting, if really accurate information were available to us, to plot a graph showing the ordinary folk's pattern of meat-eating in Scotland through the centuries. Presumably it would start off high, in the early days of sparse population and unlimited hunting opportunities; fall to an all-time low—at least for the majority—in poverty-stricken mediaeval times and later; remain low till at least the mid eighteenth century; then begin to climb slowly, to reach eventually the generally high levels of today, with steep drops for the two world wars.

It need scarcely be added that the pattern showed wide variation throughout the country. While in many areas, notably in the Highlands and Islands, meat remained until the nineteenth century, a luxury reserved principally for weddings and baptisms, the *Statistical Account* shows that this was far from being true of all. With the generally improving standards of the latter half of the eighteenth century, it is clear that butchermeat was at last beginning to reach the tables of the weavers and other better-paid workers in the Lowlands. 'All classes of workers live better now than they did formerly', we read in the report for Kilbarchan, in Renfrewshire. 'About 20 years ago tea and butcher's meat were very seldom tasted by any of the lower ranks. Now they are more or less used by people of every description.'[26] And the writer of the Cambuslang (Lanarkshire) report contrasts the year 1750, when 'little butcher's meat was consumed, and only gentlemen farmers killed their fat cattle', with the year 1791 when 'a great deal of butcher's meat is consumed'.[27] In view of its being one of the large cattle trysts, it is perhaps only to be expected that Crieff should have had ready access to meat:

> There is here a weekly market for all kinds of butcher's meat, poultry, butter, cheese, etc. Of the first article, there is ten times more sold now than 20 years ago; each kind too was then to be got only in its most plentiful season, pork in winter, veal in spring, lamb early in summer, mutton from the middle of summer to Christmas, beef from Lammas to Candlemas, when it almost totally disappeared for six months. Now that article never fails. . . . [28]

In the crofting areas at least, however, the usual practice was for a number of families to club together to buy an animal which would be divided up evenly and then pickled for (strictly limited) winter use. The salted carcases of cattle fattened for slaughter at Martinmas (11 November and a term day in Scotland) were known as marts: goats, sheep, deer and even seabirds could of course become marts as well in the areas in which they were available. Salted meat (and heavily salted at that, by all reports) was the order of the day until the mid eighteenth century at least—the actual date again showing wide variations—when, as we noted earlier, the introduction of turnips and sown grasses enabled farmers to keep far more cattle alive during the winter, so that with gradually increasing prosperity an occasional welcome feast of fresh meat began to enliven the winter menus.

Despite the paucity of meat in our ancestors' diet, it is evident that Scotland has always been a producer of beef. Thomas

Pennant, for example, noted when touring the Highlands in 1769: 'The great produce of Lochaber is cattle; that district alone sends out annually 3,000 head; but if a portion of Invernesshire is included, the number is 10,000.'[29] A considerable part of our earlier history, indeed, seems to revolve around cattle, not so much their production, it has to be admitted, as their abduction—from one glen to another; from the Lowlands to the Highlands; from the North of England across the Border. It has often been claimed, no doubt with truth, that for many of our ancestors cattle-reiving held a well-nigh irresistible appeal, providing an outlet for their sense of adventure and seemingly unquenchable thirst for raids and forays.

But one change among the many in the eighteenth century was from this illegal sport to the more peaceable trade of cattle-droving. And since the drovers, travelling slowly with large herds of beasts to the great trysts at Crieff and Falkirk, often over wild tracts of country, clearly required initiative, knowledge and endurance far beyond the ordinary, it is not surprising that this hardy breed of men came to play an important and colourful part in the Scottish scene of the eighteenth and nineteenth centuries.

In the early centuries cattle were certainly far more important than sheep, which were in fact kept more for the sake of the ewes' milk than for either mutton or wool. After sheep were widely introduced by Highland landlords, however, mutton became a much commoner item in the diet of Scotland, so that by the end of the nineteenth century the barrel of salted mutton for winter use very often took its place in the cottar houses beside the barrel of salt herrings.

Pork, known as 'poor man's beef', would certainly have been eaten occasionally. However, although the rearing of pigs had become more widespread after the advent of potatoes as a field crop, their flesh was regarded by some with distaste. In his notes on *Waverley*, Sir Walter Scott says:

> Pork, or swine's flesh, in any shape, was, till of late years, much abominated by the Scotch, nor is it yet [1814] a favourite food among them. King Jamie carried this prejudice to England, and is known to have abominated pork almost as much as he did tobacco.[30]

More commonly, this prejudice has been attributed not to the whole of Scotland but only to the Highlanders. It is interesting to note, all the same, their willingness for others to eat the offending meat, for some bred pigs and marketed them in Lowland towns. Captain Burt, commenting from the Highlands in the early eighteenth century, offers a sad reflection on the people's poverty when he observes:

I own I never saw any Swine among the Mountains, and there is good Reason for it: these People have no Offal wherewith to feed them; and were they to give them any other Food, one single Sow would devour all the Provisions of a Family.[31]

Among the common folk, venison does not appear to have played any important part apart, of course, from the great hunting days of the early centuries, and then again in more recent times in the Highlands. It was, however, available at the inns; and one wonders how well it was cooked, particularly on reading such comments as that made by Thomas Pennant on his visit to Kinloch-leven:[32] 'Breakfast on most excellent minced stag, the only form I thought that animal good in.'

It is tempting to think that, in those early days of scarcity of meat, rabbits would surely have provided a much needed source; but this clearly was not so. Although 'lords and lairds' had been directed in the seventeenth century to make 'cunningaries' (rabbit warrens), the *Statistical Account* reveals that even in the late eighteenth century rabbits could still be something of a rarity. The writer of the Dunkeld account considers his local warren worthy of special note.[33] 'There is a rabbit warren in this parish,' he writes. 'It is in a low sandy haugh, two miles to the Westward of Dunkeld. . . . On an average, 125 dozen were killed by the tacksman yearly. The skins may be valued at 6s. the dozen, and the body sells at the rate of 5d. per pair.' By the end of the following century, they were obviously in fairly common use, and in Orkney for example formed part of the farm-workers' wages. They had even become so much of a pest in some areas that the Ground Game [Hares and Rabbits] Act was passed in 1880, giving tenants the right to destroy them. Hares were used as food from quite early times, and we read of rennin from the stomachs of leverets being used in cheese-making in the Highlands. On the island of Coll it seems to have been the other way round. James Boswell notes in his Journal: 'There is a rabbit warren on the northeast of the island. . . . Young Coll intends to get some hares, of which there are none at present.'[34] Goats' flesh was another occasional source of meat in some parts, although it is clear that these animals were kept principally for their milk.

F. Marian McNeill, in her ever-popular *The Scots Kitchen,* concludes a comprehensive description of that peculiarly Scottish article, the haggis, with the suggestion that 'the use of the paunch of the animal as a receptacle of the ingredients gives that touch of romantic barbarism so dear to the Scottish heart.'[35] This may well be true. But what of the non-Scottish heart? Why is it that this, of all Scottish dishes, should have so caught the imagination not only of tourists but of countless others who have never set foot on Scottish soil? In the eighteenth century, on the contrary, it was sheep's head which enjoyed the greatest popularity: sheep's head clubs flourished as part of the fashionable Edinburgh scene, while jellied sheep's head, as a court dish, dates back to several centuries earlier. (And this to the present writer is totally incomprehensible, for the very smell of sheep's head broth remembered from childhood is still sufficient to recall distinct nausea.)

Perhaps we ourselves helped to put haggis firmly on the map, with our tall tales of hunting this elusive 'animal' with the specially-adapted legs? Be that as it may, there is little doubt that haggis, with its main ingredients liver, heart, suet and oatmeal, is well able to hold its own nutritionally with the national dishes of all other countries. (An amusing memory returns at this point of a young scientist working in the South, and presumably spurred on by the taunts of his colleagues, who presented a paper to the Nutrition Society, proving with the help of a masterly series of slides—and with a deadpan expression throughout—that our national meal of haggis, turnips and potatoes ranks second to none in the entire world.) The humble haggis, born of the ingenuity of a people perforce determined not to waste a scrap of their precious food, seems to be here to stay—plastic skin and all.

Looking at the use made of a slaughtered beast shows us our forefathers' thrift at its best. The day an ox, sheep or pig was killed would have been a red-letter day—and not exactly idle either. The head and feet made into broths and potted hough; the intestines used for holding black and white mealy puddings; the stomach stuffed to become haggis, or eaten as tripe; the meat salted in a tub for later use; the liver eaten first and the heart and lights next, with some set aside for haggis; the blood incorporated in black puddings; the suet reserved for mealy puddings and for candles; the hides kept for mats and coverings; the pigs' bristles used for making ropes to tether horses, or to collect birds' eggs on the cliffs. How altogether different from the wasteful habits of modern society!

VEGETABLES AND FRUIT

The answer to the question as to which vegetables were cultivated by our earlier ancestors is short and simple—practically none. Although it is known that a number of vegetables—peas, onions and leeks among them—were introduced to Britain by the Romans, these seem to have disappeared for many centuries, even in England, which was always ahead of Scotland in this respect. From the fifteenth century onwards, a single vegetable is mentioned over and over again: so much a part of the folk life is it, indeed, that it is found in song, story and proverb, and it alone, apart from certain wild plants, provided a slender bulwark against scurvy. That vegetable was kail.

'I was told at Aberdeen,' wrote Dr Johnson, 'that the people learned from Cromwell's soldiers to make shoes and to plant kail. How they lived without kail, it is not easy to guess: they cultivate hardly any other plant for common tables, and when they had not kail, they probably had nothing.'[36]

The poorest of cottars, we find, had their kail-yards. The precious plant could not be grown in fields because of the depredations of livestock, and it was not unusual for a kail-yard to be made out of the walls of a derelict house once the timber had been removed. Kail was used in a variety of ways. Most commonly it was incorporated, along with barley, in the ever-present broths to which our ancestors were so partial; it could also be boiled along with oatmeal, or simply served on its own, with butter and milk added when these were available. Certainly if there had to be just one winter vegetable, it was as well that it happened to be an extremely nutritious one: as a rich source of both minerals and vitamins, it had a great deal to commend it.

Until the eighteenth century, that era of maximum change, the only other cultivated vegetable of note to which the ordinary rural folk had access was cabbage—again said to have been introduced by Cromwell's troops—which generally replaced kail during the summer. In the Highlands, both of these became known relatively late, and eventually came to take the place of the common nettle in the diet of the poorer people.

In an earlier chapter we noted some of the revolutionary changes, both in agricultural practice and in diet, to which the advent of the turnip and the potato gave rise when, around the turn of the eighteenth century, they ceased to be cultivated only in the gardens of the rich and became a field crop. Yet again a look at the *Statistical Account* serves to highlight not only the significance of these changes but also the speed with which they spread all over the country. 'Ten years ago', reads the entry for Symington (Lanarkshire), which is typical of many accounts, 'there were no turnips to be seen; and now, everyone who is not doing more or less in that way, is considered as void of all spirit and skill.'[37] Turnips actually

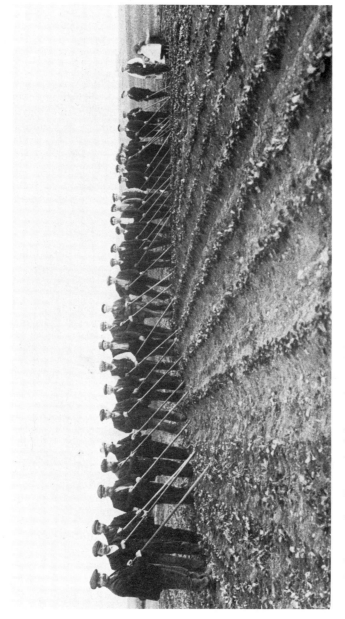

9 Hoeing match at Rango in Orkney, about 1923. Per Mrs Moar, Nisthouse, Stenness. *Source* National Museum of Antiquities of Scotland, C12194.

played their most important role in agriculture and stock-raising by making possible winter feeding of cattle and a new crop rotation; that they also enriched the rural diet by providing a reliable winter source of the valuable vitamin C, goes without saying.

An almost unprecedented contribution to the diet of the poor, however, was made by the potato. 'The potatoe is the true root of scarcity, which promises to set famine at defiance', is the bold claim made by the writer of one Perthshire report. 'The poorer sort of people dine and sup chiefly on potatoes, in the season of them.' Interestingly, though, he adds: 'But those that are in a state of servitude, are commonly above eating potatoes.'[38] Misguided snobbery indeed. Varying estimates of the extent to which potatoes figured in the daily diet of the poor are made in the report, but the one for Cadder (Lanarkshire) has it that 'potatoes are a substitute for bread, among the lower classes of people, for at least 10 months of the year'.[39]

In James T Calder (1887) we read:

> Potatoes were introduced into the county about the year 1754, and for some years after were cultivated only in the gardens of the better classes. From 1760 till 1786 the tenantry planted a few of them annually in what were called 'lazy beds'. Regarding this valuable esculent there is the following curious note in Chambers' *Traditions of Edinburgh*: 'There was long a prejudice in Scotland against the potato for two reasons—1st, That it was a species of the night-shade; 2nd, That it was a provocative to incontinence'.[40]

Writing in the nineteenth century, Osgood Mackenzie makes the great value of the potato very clear:

> There is no doubt that the people of the west coast went through periods of terrible hunger, in what we now speak of as 'the good old times', especially before the introduction of the potato. How they lived in pre-potato days is a mystery. But even prior to the destruction caused by the potato blight, when the potatoes usually grew so well, there was hardly a year in which my grandfather and my father did not import cargoes of oatmeal to keep the people alive, and those cargoes were seldom, if ever, paid for by their poor recipients.[41]

Exactly when the carrot arrived in the gardens of the poor is not altogether easy to establish; because of its outstandingly high content of the scarce vitamin A, however, its coming must have led to a further improvement in health. One can almost say for certain that by the early nineteenth century the majority of rural dwellers would have had access not only to kail, cabbage, turnips and

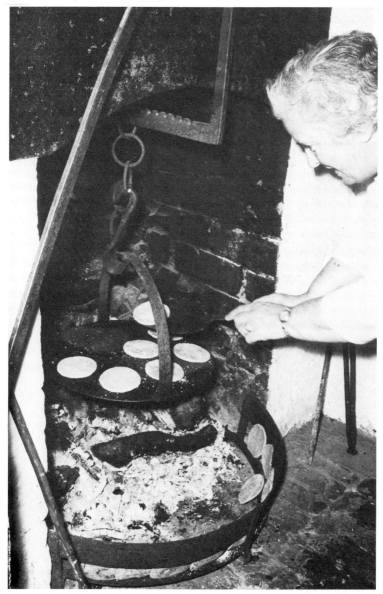

10   Baking on an open hearth, Glenesk, Angus. Photograph Alexander
Fenton. *Source* National Museum of Antiquities of Scotland,
III/51/12.

potatoes, but also to carrots, peas, beans, leeks and onions, advances in the standards of cottage gardening being in large measure due to the worthy efforts of the various agricultural and horticultural societies, although we read also of many landlords who gave an inspiring lead to their tenants.

Even in isolated places the new knowledge was being put to good use, though not, as we have already noted, without a certain amount of opposition. Dr Johnson's observation on his visit to the island of Coll (1773) is of interest in this respect:

> Young Coll, who has a very laudable desire of improving his patrimony, purposes some time to plant an orchard; which, if it be sheltered by a wall, may perhaps succeed. He has introduced the culture of turnips, of which he has a field, where the whole work was performed by his own hand. His intention is to provide food for his cattle in the winter. This innovation was considered by Mr Macsewyn as the idle project of a young head, heated with English fancies; but he has now found that turnips will really grow, and that hungry sheep and cows will really eat them.[42]

The gardens of the upper classes had always produced a reasonable variety of vegetables; we find that by the early nineteenth century this included not only those listed above, but also the rarer tomatoes and lettuces, as well as broccoli, endives, celery, artichokes and cauliflower. And of this last we find an interesting mention, in that 'colliflower' appeared on the menu of an Edinburgh Corporation dinner as early as 1703.

There can surely be few articles of food which have actually come down in price since the eighteenth century. Nevertheless, this does seem to have happened with rhubarb, that very common root which we take for granted today. In the *Statistical Account* for Dunkeld we read this intriguing comment:

> In 1770, some seeds of the RHEUM PALMATUM were sent from Peterburgh, by Dr Mounsey, to His Grace [the Duke of Atholl]. They were planted, and considerable attention was paid to the culture of that root. Rhubarb, to the value of £160 sterling, was sold in one season, to a London druggist, at the rate of 8s. the lb. In short, full proof was afforded, that rhubarb may be raised and dressed in Britain, equal in all its qualities, to what is now, at so high a price, imported from the East Indies and from Russia and Turkey.[43]

This highly successful business venture may, for all we know, have been repeated in many other places; in any case the root, valued mainly for its known aperient qualities, was to be found within a century in most cottage gardens.

As to the cultivation of fruit in Scotland, its story takes even less time to tell than that of vegetables. Neither the soil nor the climate being generally suitable for the growing of fruit, this important food was virtually absent from the ordinary Scots' diet until at least the mid eighteenth century. One of the many beneficial changes of that era was the very gradual appearance in cottage gardens of black currants, red currants, and gooseberries (which up to this time had been confined to the gardens of the gentry) with doubtless, concomitant good effects on the general standards of health. By the end of the nineteenth century the making of jams and jellies had obviously become a recognised part of the traditional rural work-cycle. By that time, too, the soft fruits industry was becoming well-established—strawberries in Clydesdale, raspberries in Perthshire—much of which fruit eventually reached the jam factories of Dundee. A new, sweet food had arrived on the Scottish tea-table.

A few places had proved to be admirably suited to the growing of hard fruits: these were for the most part in the Lowlands, particularly the upper Clyde valley. Clearly there were other locations, notably the fertile county of Moray, as well as some coastal areas where the benign influence of the Gulf Stream doubtless played its part. Osgood Mackenzie refers, for example, to the plentiful supply of peaches, nectarines, plums and cherries to which as a child he had access on the family estates in Ross-shire, as well as to 'hundreds of sacks of [hazel] nuts, every one full to the neck, sent in cartloads to the Beauly markets'.[44]

The Lanarkshire reports in the *Statistical Account* are particularly illuminating. In that for Carluke we read that 'fruit abounds more in this parish, than anywhere in the Clyde, or even in Scotland'.[45] The orchards do not, however, appear to have enjoyed unqualified success. 'There are a good many little orchards,' reads the entry for Hamilton, 'producing apples, pears, plums and cherries. In good seasons, they bear very good and well-flavoured fruit, but there is scarcely one year in three, in which the orchards turn to good account. . . . Considerable quantities of gooseberries and currants, produced here, are sent to the Glasgow market.'[46] As far north as the Carse of Gowrie, too, the orchards were reaching their peak of productivity during the late eighteenth and early nineteenth centuries, although sadly they declined thereafter, due, it has been claimed, to insufficient attention to their cultivation.

It would seem safe to assume that by the late eighteenth century some fruit was at last reaching the poorer folk, although again it has to be added that this was true principally in Lowland areas. For the rich, of course, fruit had long been available. Dried fruits are known to have been imported as early as Mary Queen of Scots' reign; oranges and lemons began to appear more than a century later. With increasing knowledge of cultivation, too, the gentry's gardens are known to have been producing a surprisingly wide variety by the end of the eighteenth century. 'In the gardens of Carstairs House, which are extensive,' reads the entry for Carstairs, in Lanarkshire, 'not only the fruits that are common, but grapes, pine apples, melons and everything which the country can produce in this way, are raised in great abundance. The tea, coffee and other plants have been tried and thrive beyond expectation.'[47]

In considering the obviously deficient supply of fruit and vegetables in the common people's diet prior to the eighteenth century, we should study the extent to which use was made of wild plants. There is indeed much evidence that many were used, although knowledge in this field is limited. It is known that wild fruits such as raspberries, brambles, blaeberries and in some areas cloudberries were eaten, but less is known about elderberries and cranberries, although the former have been popular for wine-making for many centuries. We noted already (see Chapter 3) mention of the use of 'watercresses, sloes, hawthorns, hipthorns, hazelnuts, crab apples'. Burt makes one brief comment on this subject:

> The only Fruit the Natives have, that I have seen, is the bilberry, much esteemed by the inhabitants, who eat them with their Milk; yet in the Mountain-Woods, which for the most Part are distant and difficult of Access, there are Nuts, Raspberries, and Strawberries . . . but those Woods are so rare, that few of the Highlanders are near enough to partake of their Benefit.[48]

In the Highlands at least the use of young nettles—a good source of vitamin C—continued into the nineteenth century and in some cases into the present century. Also mentioned earlier were wild spinach (in Gaelic *blionigean*), wild garlic and wild carrots; as well as earthnuts and various types of seaweed, in particular carrageen which is popular to this day. Special mention should be made of silverweed (*potentilla anserina*), known in Gaelic as *brisgean*. A creeping plant which grows on the shingle, it is familiar to all who frequent the Hebridean *machair*. It is clear that the root of this plant was much used in times of scarcity, being dried and ground into meal for making porridge and even a kind of bread. In *Carmina Gadelica* an extraordinary claim is made for the plant:

> The root was much used throughout the Highlands and Islands before the potato was introduced. It was cultivated, and grew to a consider-

able size. A man could sustain himself on a square of ground his own length.[49]

Martin Martin visiting St Kilda around the year 1695, mentions the use of sorrel leaves—and at the same time gives the earliest account of a weight-reducing diet known to the present writer.

> One of them that was become corpulent, and had his throat almost shut up, being advised by me to take salt with his meat, to exercise himself more in the fields than he had done of late, to forbear eating of fat fowl and the fat pudding called giben, and to eat sorrel, was very much concerned because all this was very disagreeable, and my advising him to eat sorrel perfectly a surprise to him; but when I bid him consider how the fat fulmar eat this plant he was at last disposed to take my advice; and by this means alone in few days after, his voice was much clearer, his appetite recovered, and he was in a fair way of recovery.[50]

It need hardly be said that the whole topic of fruit and vegetable consumption revolves around scurvy, the dread spectre of which hung over the people of Scotland for centuries, although obviously it receded significantly after the introduction of the turnip and potato. We do know, however, that a serious outbreak occurred at the time of the potato famine in 1845 and 1846. In this respect the most interesting question concerns rose-hips, our countryside's phenomenally rich source of vitamin C. To what extent, if at all, did our ancestors eat these? As country children have always tended to nibble them, one might surmise that this has always been the case—an important point, since it would be true to say that a rose-hip a day would have kept the scurvy away. It is possible that somebody might have died of that disease while rose-hips grew at his doorstep.

Pursuing the subject in the *Statistical Account,* it is intriguing to try to discover whether any connection was made between the incidence of scurvy and the growing of vegetables. Obviously there must have been some areas in which vegetables simply did not grow well. The entry for Blackford, Perthshire, gives cause for reflection:

> The soil in this parish is not good: the effects of the cold are sensibly felt in retarding and marring the growth of vegetables. Most of the diseases, which take their rise from a cold damp air, prevail here, such as rheums and pulmonary complaints: but the scurvy is the most prevalent disease; and is attended by violent symptoms, such as aching pains in the joints and limbs, and hard livid swellings. In some cases

tumours are formed, which suppurate and degenerate into scrofulous runnings: in some instances it affects the judgment, and makes the unhappy sufferers put an end to their own existence.[51]

We may add that the unfortunate victims were also likely to have sore, bleeding mouths and to lose their teeth, and to suffer from haemorrhages as well.

The concept of deficiency diseases is familiar today. But it is clear from our ancestors' writings that in their estimation diseases were caused *by* some agent, never because of something being absent. An example from the account for the parish of Arngask, Perthshire, illustrates this point: 'The scurvy is likewise a common disorder, which originates as is supposed, from the too frequent use of oatmeal.'[52] Consider too the entry for Hamilton:

> The scurvy is almost unknown, though oatmeal makes a great part of the food of the people. Those who are disposed to reprobate the use of this wholesome and nourishing fund of subsistence, ought to examine the healthy and blooming countenances of the people in this country, who feed on scarcely any other food, before they condemn the use of it in toto.[53]

The intriguing question as to what might have been included under the heading of 'scarcely any other food' is unfortunately not answered.

In 1747 the Scots naval surgeon James Lind carried out the experiment which was later to become famous as the first controlled clinical trial. 'On the 20th of May 1747,' wrote Lind, 'I took 12 patients in the scurvy, on board the Salisbury at sea. They all in general had putrid gums, the spots and lassitude, with weakness of their knees.'[54] He then described the various supplements given to the sailors—vinegar, elixir vitriol, sea-water, cider—as well as that prescribed for the two lucky ones, which was two oranges and one lemon per day.

> The consequence was that the most sudden and visible good effects were perceived from the use of the oranges and lemons; one of those who had taken them, being at the end of six days fit for duty . . . the other was the best recovered of any in his condition, and being now deemed pretty well, was appointed nurse to the rest of the sick.

In 1782 another naval surgeon, Charles Curtis, quoted the advice of a certain 'Mr Young of the Navy':

> Nothing is more necessary for the cure of this disease in any situation where there is tolerably pure air, than not dead and dried, but a fresh

vegetable diet, of greens and roots, in sufficient quantity. To be sure, we cannot have a kitchen garden at sea.[55]

In view of these findings the most intriguing question of all is just how long it took for the news to percolate through to the doctors in the rural areas of Scotland, to say nothing of the ordinary folk? Would sailors have passed it on to their families? Perhaps we should bear in mind that it took till 1804, about half a century after Dr Lind published his *Treatise of the Scurvy*, for the Royal Navy to end this scourge by supplying sailors with lime juice. The trouble was that even if news of the efficacy of citrus fruits did become common knowledge, these fruits would be beyond the reach of the ordinary folk.

The Household Books of some of Scotland's great houses, as we have seen already, can at times furnish fascinating glimpses into their life and times. A snippet from one such book of accounts provides us with a most interesting anecdote, and indeed a heart-warming note on which this section may fittingly be ended. Among the entries for January 1773 it is noticeable that there are several for considerable quantities of oranges and lemons. In explanation, the writer has added this footnote: 'A fever raged at the time for which Dr Farquharson prescribed lemons and oranges among the sick people's drink, and as they were all very poor, the fruit was furnished to them out of the Castle.' All honour to the unknown Dr Farquharson, not only for his knowledge but, presumably, for his powers of persuasion—and to the owners of the Castle for such a generous response.

BEVERAGES

Apart from milk in its various forms—buttermilk, fresh milk, whey— and ordinary spring water, the principal drink of the common folk of Scotland until the eighteenth century was ale. Heather ale was used in some areas: Pennant mentions it, for example, as having been made in Islay. But the ale in common use was brewed from barley and oats. Ale is mentioned, indeed, long before whisky, which does not appear until the fifteenth century. Wine was by no means unknown: the early native variety was made by fermenting the liquid tapped from birch trees, and in mediaeval times foreign wines were imported in exchange for Scotland's exports of wool, hides and fish. These, however, were generally beyond the reach of ordinary people.

It was not until 1725, when Parliament brought in the Malt Tax (6*d*. on every bushel of malt) that the rise in the price of 'twopenny' ale had the effect of greatly increasing whisky-drinking in Scotland. And a most unpopular tax it was. Henry Graham writes:

> Ale had been made in every farm, manse, and mansion. At this tyrannical interference with their favourite drink the people arose in wild indignation. There were fierce riots in Glasgow; Edinburgh brewers refused to brew so long as the hateful impost lasted, thus promising to deprive all citizens of their drink and bakers of the yeast to make the daily bread; and certainly from that year the brewing of 'twopenny' steadily declined, effectively to make way for the more potent drink of whisky, which was then almost unknown.[56]

Many of the writers in the *Statistical Account* bewail the substitution of whisky for the more wholesome ale. In the Glasgow report we read:

> It is to be lamented that by the cheapness of spiritous liquors, and the increasing use of them, many young people of both sexes are easily corrupted and ruined. Happy would it be . . . if fewer public-houses were licensed, the use of spiritous liquors checked, and good wholesome ale substituted in their place.[57]

Certainly there would seem to have been no scarcity of public-houses, even in country places. There is a strangely modern ring about the entry for Carnwath (Lanarkshire):

> There are six public-houses in the village, in which small beer, porter, but particularly whisky, are sold; and it is to be regretted that this last article should be so cheap, as it is evidently tending to debauch the morals of the lower classes. The quantity consumed here is almost incredible; and those who are least able to spare from their families are most addicted to this abominable beverage.[58]

Owing to its cheapness and, presumably, the ease with which it could be home-produced, a very considerable amount of whisky must have been drunk after 1725. Excessive drinking was clearly a feature of Scottish life—for the common folk, mainly upon occasions such as births and deaths, and perhaps especially at those feasts known as Penny Bridals, at which anyone who could afford a penny seems to have been welcome to drink copiously of the 'braithel ale' freely provided. Wherever conditions of harshness and squalor prevail, a degree of intemperance is surely not to be wondered at; such an explanation, however, perhaps fails to account for the vast popularity of gentlemen's clubs in the cities, establishments not exactly distinguished for their sobriety.

Dr Johnson observed no drunkenness in the people of the Western Isles:

> A man of the Hebrides, for of the woman's diet I can give no account, as soon as he appears in the morning, swallows a glass of whisky; yet they are not a drunken race, at least I never was present at much intemperance; but no man is so abstemious as to refuse the morning dram, which they call a 'skalk'.[59]

Yet, however acute in his observations, Dr Johnson was a tourist in Scotland, and it might thus be more valid to take note of what a resident in the Highlands has to say of its people's drinking habits. Elizabeth Grant seems to have few doubts about the over-indulgence prevalent on Speyside in her time (around 1800):

> The whisky was a bad habit. At every house it was offered; at every house it must be tasted or offence would be given. I am sure that had we steadily refused compliance with so incorrect a custom it would have been far better for ourselves, and might sooner have put an end to so pernicious a habit among the people. Whisky-drinking was and is the bane of the country: from early morning till late at night it went on.

But she does then add a postscript in extenuation:

> All the men engaged in the wood manufacture drank it in goblets three times a day, yet except at a merry-making we never saw anyone tipsy.[60]

As far as nutrition is concerned, we may suppose that for men working long, hard hours in the fields or forests, a much-needed addition to their energy intake must have been supplied in this way.

For the upper classes in Scotland, claret remained the firm favourite until at least the eighteenth century. In Edinburgh it was wheeled in casks around the streets; its popularity began to wane, however, with the ending of free imports at the end of that century.

There is a brief but interesting snippet in Boswell's Diary showing the selection of beverages one could expect in a gentleman's house of the day. Of the meal which he and Dr Johnson enjoyed as guests of Captain Macdonald of Kingsburgh, in Skye, and his wife, the former Miss Flora Macdonald, he says:

> As genteel a supper as one would wish to see, in particular an excellent roasted turkey, porter to drink at table, and after supper claret and punch.[61]

Having mentioned the celebrated Flora, it is of at least equal interest to read of Bonnie Prince Charlie's very different kind of experience while a fugitive, and disguised, in the inn at Portree. Eric Linklater writes in *The Prince in the Heather*:

> Unwilling, as it seems, to open his bottle of brandy, he enquired what drink there was in the inn. Only whisky or water he was told; for in all the Isle of Skye beer and ale were to be found only in gentlemen's houses. He asked for milk, but there was none. He must drink water, said Donald Roy, and offered him an ugly vessel that the innkeeper used for bailing out his boat. He had just drunk from it himself, and when he saw the Prince look doubtfully at it he whispered—for the innkeeper was in the room—that he must not show untimely delicacy for fear of arousing suspicion. So the Prince took a hearty draught.[62]

And what of St Kilda, the most remote outpost of all? In 1695 Martin Martin wrote:

> Their drink is water, or whey, commonly. They brew ale but rarely, using the juice of nettleroots, which they put in a dish with a little barley-meal dough; these sowens (i.e. flummery) being blended together, produce good yeast, which puts their wort [pre-fermentation liquor] into a ferment, and makes good ale, so that when they drink plentifully of it, it disposes them to dance merrily.[63]

During the eighteenth century another drink apart from whisky was taking the place of ale, one which might have been thought harmless enough, but which in fact seems to have aroused more general spleen than that occasioned by whisky. That drink was, of course, tea. So far as is known, it was introduced towards the end of the seventeenth century, and at first its correct use seems to have been a mystery to many, some ladies for example offering the tea-leaves to visitors on buttered bread. Graham writes:

> The fashion of tea-drinking, becoming common about 1720, had to make its way against fierce opposition. The patriotic condemned tea as a foreign drink hurtful to national industry; the old-fashioned protested against it as a new-fangled folly; the robust scorned it as an effeminate practice; magistrates and energetic laymen put it in the same malignant category as smuggled spirits.[64]

But despite, or perhaps because of, all this antagonism, it becomes apparent that within a few decades the ladies have been won over and are in no way reluctant to leave the gentlemen to their port and repair to their 'dish of tea'. The afternoon tea meal begins to be surrounded with great elegance, not to mention many baked dainties, and the Scottish afternoon teas become, among the wealthier classes at least, as famous as their sumptuous breakfasts.

Tea was at first obviously a luxury, but as its price gradually fell, and as living standards began slowly to rise during the eighteenth century, the common people too began to develop a taste for the new, fashionable beverage. The *Statistical Account* for Crieff reads:

> Above twenty times more tea is used now than 20 years ago. Bewitched by the mollifying influence of an enfeebling potion, the very poorest classes begin to regard it as one of the necessaries of life, and for its sake resign the cheaper and more invigorating nourishment which the productions of this country afford.[65]

Does the writer here refer to milk or ale?

Tea had come to stay, however. By the nineteenth century it had found its way into the humblest of dwellings. 'In 1778', runs another report, 'there were not four houses in the parish where tea was drunk; now (1798) it is used in every house'. High tea became established as the evening meal in the farming community; the tea-room, too, soon arrived. And it has to be said that the era of Scotland's addiction to carbohydrate foods had begun in earnest.

SUGAR AND SWEET FOODS

In early times, honey, first that of wild bees and later of the cultivated variety, was the only sweet food known to our ancestors. One contributor to the *Statistical Account* waxes lyrical on the subject of honey and bees:

> Several persons in this parish have propagated bees with great success. The numerous orchards, the extensive plantations of trees, which abound with the saccharine juice, the large fields of beans, whose grateful flavour embalms the very air in the Carse, and the uplands adorned with variegated blossoms of clover and daisies, and furze and broom, afford a plentiful supply to these industrious insects.[66]

Although it did not come into general use until the eighteenth and nineteenth centuries, it seems fairly clear that the Scots had fallen under the spell of sugar, and especially 'sweeties', a great deal earlier.

In the Middle Ages, sugar was both scarce and dear; and while we do read of kists of sugar being included in cargoes from Holland by the end of the fourteenth century, their destination was either the apothecaries' shops, where the sugar would be incorporated into medicines, or else the houses of the wealthy. Records show, however, that on gala occasions in Edinburgh sweets were distributed to the eager populace, some of the delicacies mentioned including scrozats, carmis and succatis (these last being sugar-coated nuts or orange pips).

Following the establishment in the seventeenth century of the East India Company, cane sugar began to be cheaper and somewhat easier to come by. Beet sugar made its appearance in the eighteenth century, and it was then too that the back-street sweetie-shop began to be a feature of many Scots towns and cities. The peculiarly Scots tablet (fudge elsewhere) without which no church sale is to this day complete, is known to have been on sale in Edinburgh's streets during the eighteenth century; then, too, such favourites as bull's-eyes, liquorice, peppermint drops and Gibraltar rock ('jib') were popular. By the nineteenth century the repertoire included many more, for example acid drops, humbugs and Conversation Lozenges. The number of sweetie-shops Scotland was able to support began to be a source of amazement to foreign visitors, and many towns became known as much for their confectionery as for their shortbread, cakes, bridies, or biscuits.

Although the sweet trade flourished mainly in the towns, pedlars also dispensed confections in country places. One of these pedlars, a familiar figure around Kelso in the Borders towards the end of the nineteenth century, is commemorated in the song Coulter's Candy. Of its many verses, with seemingly endless variations, the most interesting to the student of diet is the one which shows, a little surprisingly perhaps, that the connection between sweets and increasing girth was well recognised:

> Puir wee Jeanie she was gettin' awfu' thin
> A rickle o' banes covered ower wi' skin;
> Noo she's gettin' a wee double chin
> Wi' sookin' Coulter's Candy.

Interestingly, the early Scots reputation for sweets rested solely upon the boiled sugar variety: the more expensive chocolate was used in liquid form until slab chocolate began to be used in the latter part of the nineteenth century.

Black treacle was one derivative of sugar which the poor people in Scotland did have; its high content of calcium and iron made it a food of some considerable value. Around 1900 it began to be displaced by the sweeter but less nourishing golden syrup, which continues to be the favourite to this day.

Few would disagree that the advent of cheap sugar, bringing in its wake a host of sugar-based products—commercially prepared jams of inferior quality, sweets, cakes, and biscuits—which eventually penetrated via the ubiquitous vans even to the furthest Highlands and Islands, heralded for the Scots diet a decidedly retrograde step. In later chapters we shall be taking a look at some of the health problems to which this eventually gave rise.

5

THE 'PURE, NATURAL FOOD' OF DAYS GONE BY

Was it really like this?

'Pure food' enthusiasts have been around for a long time. Not, it may be added, in any great numbers; for this enthusiasm is surely a preserve of the privileged, the already adequately fed, who can afford to be selective. The more pressing problem for a great many of our ancestors in Scotland, as for many millions in the world today, was how to stay alive at all. This having been said, however, our own history clearly shows the debt we owe to those who campaigned, often at great personal risk, for good-quality, uncontaminated food. Perhaps this can best be illustrated by looking at the history of bread, that staple food of Western man from time immemorial.

In the ancient civilisations, notably of Greece and Rome, wheat ground between large stones produced a flour of darkish hue which went to make the bread of the poorer folk. A much whiter flour could be made, however, by successive sievings—an expensive process which meant that the rich could have white (and incidentally, less nutritious) bread, thereafter inevitably to be associated with wealth and prestige. But another attitude can also be discerned, and this is where the 'natural food' bias would seem to begin, in that many of the classical writers saw brown bread as symbolising the wholesome simplicity of country life; and to some extent this predominantly intellectual viewpoint may be seen to have survived the centuries and given rise to the 'health foods' boom of today.

These conflicting attitudes can be traced right through mediaeval times in England. Wheat continued to be ground between large stones, often by water-power; and while most of the flour was of high extraction rate, again whiter flour could be produced and was bought by the rich. In Scotland, as we saw earlier, the situation was different. Oats and barley provided the bulk of the bread—or more accurately, bannocks—until, in the urban areas at least, wheaten bread began to take over towards the end of the eighteenth century.

On three separate occasions (1756–8, 1772–4 and 1795–1800) Parliament authorised the sale of a browner loaf, but although it was a penny cheaper (no mean reduction in those days), it was far from popular. The public continued to clamour for white bread. This craving led to trouble which was by no means confined to nutritional deprivation. The bakers began to add alum, a substance which not only whitened the loaf but also increased its size and improved its texture. That this might not be the only additive began to be suspected when in 1757 the anonymous author of a pamphlet entitled *Poison detected; or frightful truths and alarming to the British Metropolis* alleged that 'sacks of unground bones' were being used to increase the bulk of flour. 'The charnel houses of the dead are raked to add filthiness to the food of the living', was his macabre assertion. This turned out to be merely the first salvo in what was to be a long war, with accusations (some quite ludicrously exaggerated) being hurled at the millers and bakers, whose first reply, *Modest apology in defence of the bakers*, appeared in 1758.

It was not until the latter half of the nineteenth century that the advent of roller-mills enabled the millers to produce white flour cheaply, and incidentally to make a rattling profit on the side by selling the 'offals' as cattle fodder. So at last the city poor achieved their coveted white loaf, with predictably detrimental consequences to health, since the two most important parts of the grain, the germ and the bran, were being lost.

Robert Louis Stevenson, in *Travels with a Donkey in the Cevennes*,[1] provides a good example of prevailing attitudes about bread, both his own and that of the French peasants among whom he travelled. Writing of his purchase of the donkey which was to be his pack-animal, he tells of how her former owner 'professed himself greatly touched by the separation, and declared he had often bought white bread for the donkey when he had been content with black bread for himself; but this, according to the best authorities, must have been a flight of fancy. He had a name in the village for brutally misusing the ass; yet it is certain that he shed a tear, and the tear made a clean mark down one cheek.' R L S, however, conformed to the expected pattern: his provision list turns out to be 'a leg of cold mutton, a bottle of Beaujolais, an empty bottle to carry milk, an egg-beater, and a considerable quantity of black bread and white'. The black bread was, of course, for the donkey.

In the mid nineteenth century, the 'natural food' protagonists were engaged in a battle against the practice of whitening flour artificially by the addition of chemical bleaching agents. Although many of their number, notably Allinson in the United Kingdom and Graham in the USA, put up a spirited fight to bring back a browner, more nutritious loaf, they never did succeed in doing so. And even if they had, it is doubtful whether the ordinary folk of their day would have eaten it. In the event, it was to be about a hundred years before any actual legislation regarding the extraction rate of flour was passed in this country, and then only because of the exceptional situation brought about by the Second World War; while agene (nitrogen trichloride), the most notorious of the bleaching agents, was not finally banned until 1953.

To return, however, to the question posed in this chapter heading: was the food of former times really as pure and unadulterated as some would have us believe? The more one delves into social history, the more this myth is exposed—indeed, the scale upon which adulteration was practised is to us today wellnigh incredible. It must be stated all the same, that the story of adulterated food belongs almost exclusively, in Scotland's case, to the urban areas: the rural Scots, subsisting on their oats and barley, potatoes and kail, milk and cheese, were happily immune from this particular evil.

The tricks of the manufacturers of the day lacked little in ingenuity. We read of brick-dust added to cocoa, acorns to coffee, tallow to butter. Milk, it seems, might have chalk added, or could be sold on city streets diluted with hot water to give the impression of being warm from the cow. Tea was an especial target—used tea leaves being bought up from hotels and coffee-houses, stiffened with gum, blackened with black-lead, and sold as the real article. Or it could be 'improved' by being coloured green—to the extent that people actually preferred it so, and found genuine tea rather dull. In 1852, one tea company took the unusual step of engaging a lecturer to go round telling his audiences what tea should look like. Nor did alcoholic beverages escape either: faked wines were widely sold, and beer, gin, and cider all suffered, sometimes dangerously, from adulteration.

It is mainly to the science of chemistry that we owe the eventual exposure of malpractices regarding food, a significant example being the ability to identify the watering-down of milk, by estimation of its fat content. In 1850, thirty years after Accum, a reputable chemist, had suffered imprisonment and ruin for daring to publish *A Treatise on the adulteration of food and culinary poisons,* the *Lancet* finally set up an enquiry. Five years later, a special Commission was appointed to investigate the matter, with the result that the first Food and Drugs Act was passed in 1860, and the second in 1872.

If we are amazed at the scale of food adulteration, even as it appears in this far-from-exhaustive account, we can still perhaps understand something of what triggered it off. Sheer commercialism—or, more bluntly, greed—may have been the primary factor, but it is also true that with the excessively rapid growth of the industrial population, there arose an urgent necessity to bring into the towns and cities enough food, in a sufficiently palatable state, to feed large numbers of people. Scarcity of raw materials, lack of transport, and especially the absence of any efficient food industry, made this an impossible task.

The passing of the first Food and Drugs Acts laid the foundation of the food legislation which we have come to take for granted today. With the backing of Parliament, a system of controls has gradually evolved over the past hundred years, bringing us to the present position in which we can have a high degree of confidence in the quality of our food.

Or can we? That the whole subject of 'pure food' and especially food additives is a controversial and emotive one, few would be likely to deny. (Moreover, it is beyond both the scope of this book and the knowledge of.the present writer.) The facts may be stated very briefly on both sides of the argument, however, in the awareness that it is necessary to avoid being complacent on the one hand and alarmist on the other.

It would be wrong to give the impression that the question of food purity is taken lightly in this country. In this whole field the Ministry of Agriculture and Fisheries is responsible to Parliament: regulations concerning food additives are the concern of the Food Standards Committee, while the Medical Research Council, in conjunction with many public analysts, as well as chemists and microbiologists employed by the food manufacturers, have responsibility for ensuring our consumption of safe food.

As most are aware, there exists a list of permitted additives for food preservation (although the modern preference is, naturally, for freezing and dehydration) as well as a number of organic dyes, sweeteners and fat emulsifiers. Also, antioxidants may be added to fats and oils, and the 'improver' chlorine dioxide to flour in bread-making.

Despite all known tests and precautions, doubts still remain in the minds of many reputable health professionals. For one thing, no series of tests can in fact prove an additive safe: it is, rather, a case of weighing up the available evidence and deciding whether the benefits outweigh the risks. Nor is the fact that the permitted list of additives is not identical in every country conducive to complacency. Could it not also be said that it is a doubtful food which needs an artificial dye to secure its attractiveness? Finally, the real cause for concern today is the *extent* to which the developed world is now feeding its population on 'designed consumer foods'—that is, natural foods such as potatoes and wheat used not as foods in their own right, but as raw materials for producing new, highly processed foods, almost inevitably involving the addition of artificial colourings and flavourings. While a proportion of processed foods (after all, even bread and butter have undergone processing of a kind) may in an industrial society be considered inevitable, the considerable extent to which these are consumed by many people undoubtedly gives rise to serious questions.

If a sense of proportion is called for in the matter of 'pure food', this is surely true also in the area of so-called 'health foods'. Here things have changed vastly since the days when Allinson and Graham battled for their wholemeal loaf, and were labelled cranks for so doing. Nowadays large numbers, predominantly from the younger professional groups, buy a substantial part of their food over the counter of health or whole food stores. On the credit side, it should certainly be acknowledged that these have performed a most important service. Not only have they frequently provided items unobtainable elsewhere; they have also served to raise general standards of nutrition, most notably perhaps by increasing public awareness of the excellence of wholemeal bread and many other whole foods. On the other hand, vigilance is required in the matter of various food supplements, beguiling labels, and at times exaggerated claims, as well as unnecessarily fancy packaging: the plain, unpackaged product is often to be found in the local grain store at a much lower price.

Obviously the answer lies in sound, basic nutrition education, with resolute debunking of common fallacies; since a well-informed public will not be misled by extravagant claims. Healthy eating means a prudent choice of ordinary wholesome foods. Contrary to the belief of many, this need involve neither great expense nor unduly complicated effort. But it does involve the acquisition of basic knowledge.

Nevertheless, to become too slavishly concerned with our food—constantly worrying about whether it will 'do us good'—is surely also undesirable. While it may, like all excesses, be regarded for the most part with tolerant amusement, set against the horrifying background of world hunger, it can easily be seen in quite a different light.

An historical study, however sketchy, of 'pure' food would seem somewhat incomplete if we failed to look at the closely allied subject of 'clean' food. Here, glancing back through the centuries can at times be diverting—to those, that is, with strong stomachs. Much of our information here comes, not surprisingly, from the early visitors from South of the Border, most of whom are nothing if not frank about the unhygienic habits of our ancestors. To be fair, their attacks are aimed principally at public eating-places, presumably because these would be frequented most—and because it would have been a shade discourteous to expose their hostesses' unsavoury practices.

Captain Burt, mentioned earlier as agent and engineer in General Wade's service in the early eighteenth century, was far from enamoured of the inns in which he was sometimes obliged to eat. He describes his very first encounter with a Scottish hostelry thus:

> I asked what was to be had, and she told me potted Pigeons; and nothing, I thought, could be more agreeable, after a Day's Journey in which I had taken nothing. . . . Presently after, the Pot of Pigeons was set on the Table . . . two or three Pigeons lay mangled in the Pot, and behind were the Furrows, in the Butter, of those Fingers that had raked them out of it, and the Butter itself needed no close Application to discover its Quality. My Disgust at this Sight was so great, and being a brand-new Traveller in this Country, I ate a Crust of Bread, and drank about a pint of good Claret; and although the Night was approaching, I called for my Horses, and marched off.[2]

When we turn to look at the conditions prevailing in the towns and cities of Scotland during the eighteenth and nineteenth centuries, we find conditions in the slums that almost beggar description: those of Glasgow were considered by many to be, from the time of the Industrial Revolution onwards, the worst in Europe. In particular to some Highland families, forced to migrate to the city after being evicted from their ancient holdings, existence among these filthy surroundings might well have seemed worse than death. E Haldane in *The Scotland of our Fathers* has this to say:

> People were crowded into filthy dark cellars . . . dirt and disease were everywhere; fourteen and fifteen people occupied one room, some of them on the floor with fever. Doctors urged the removal of the dung-hills and pools of filth, and suggested paving the closes, but in vain. Wynds were often so narrow that a cart could not pass along them, and out of these opened a close or court, in the centre of which was a dunghill. Edinburgh was bad, but nothing like as bad as Glasgow.[3]

To expect anybody at all to have anything resembling clean food in such surroundings would seem to be out of the question, although one might assume that in small towns and remote hamlets the outlook would be better. In fact, Burt, living in Inverness (then a very small town), disabuses us of this idea:

> The Chasms in the Inside and Middle of these [house] Walls render them Receptacles for prodigious Numbers of Rats, which scratch their Way from the Inside of the House half through the Wall, where they burrow and breed securely . . . and such Numbers of them are seen by the Morning Twilight in the Streets, for Water, after dry Weather succeeded by a Shower of Rain, as is incredible.[4]

Small wonder that diseases like typhus, smallpox, dysentery and cholera flourished in such conditions.

Surely then, in remote village communities and especially in the islands, an altogether higher standard must have prevailed? Writings of the time do not support any such idea. The eighteenth-century French geologist Faujas de St Fond has left an interesting account of his visit to the island of Staffa and its sixteen inhabitants in 1784.[5] It happened that some others of his party were marooned on the island before Faujas arrived; when eventually they were re-united after their two-day stay in close proximity to the islanders, they entreated Faujas and the others not to come near them. 'Fly, fly from us,' they cried, 'we have brought some good specimens of mineralogy, but our collection of insects is numerous and horrible.' And little wonder: in the interval they had not only shared the hut accommodation of a woman, six children, a cow, a pig and some fowls, but had slept on some straw which had been used to litter the cow for several days before.

St Kilda was ravaged by tetanus until as recently as the 1890s. Poor hygiene may well have been the cause, since the people lived close to both their cattle and the dung-heaps. Many medicals of the day were convinced that the cause of the appallingly high infant mortality was the habit of smearing the severed umbilical cord with a mixture of dung and fulmar oil, the oil being kept in a somewhat unlikely receptacle, the stomach of a gannet. It has to be added, however, that general adherence to the above practice was never actually proved; all that can be said is that tetanus was conquered in the end by the antiseptic methods introduced by the island's minister of the time.

But, perhaps because of the sheer contrasts involved, it is our beautiful capital city which, time and time again, brings forth comments of horrified unbelief from one visitor after another to

Scotland. One wonders whether at any time, in any age or civilisation, there can have existed side by side such literary and philosophical achievement, such grandeur, snobbery and high fashion, with such appalling standards of hygiene. Burt is explicit on the subject:

> This happened to a Friend of mine. Some years ago he took a House, or Floor, within Half a Quarter of a Mile of Edinburgh, which was then about to be let by a Woman of Distinction. He immediately after her Removal, went to view his Bargain. The Floor of the Room where she saw Company was clean, being rubbed every Morning according to Custom: but the Insides of the Corner-Cupboards, and every other Part out of Sight, were in a dirty Condition but, when he came to the Kitchen, he was not only disgusted at the Sight of it, but sick with the Smell, which was intolerable; he could not so much as guess whether the Floor was Wood or Stone, it was covered so deep with accumulated Grease and Dirt, mingled together. The Drawers under the Table looked as if they were almost transparent with Grease; the Walls near the Servants' Table, which had been white, were almost covered with Snuff spit against it; and Bones of Sheep's Heads lay scattered under the Dresser. . . . Well, he hired two Women to cleanse this Augean Part, and brought a vast Quantity of Sweet-Herbs wherewith to rub it everywhere: and yet he could not bear the Smell of it a Month afterwards.[6]

But whatever the interiors of the houses were like, and they must surely have been pretty unsavoury, it is the incredible habit of flinging the household slops out of the windows which invariably catches the attention of the visitor. Nor is Captain Burt silent on this score:

> We supped very plentifully and drank good French Claret, and were very merry till the Clock struck Ten, the Hour when everybody is at Liberty, by Beat of the City Drum, to throw their Filth out at the Windows. Then the Company began to light Pieces of Paper, and throw them upon the Table to smoke the Room, and, as I thought, to mix one bad Smell with another. . . . When I was in Bed, I was forced to hide my Head between the Sheets; for the Smell of the Filth, thrown out by the Neighbours on the Back-Side of the House, came pouring into the Room to such a Degree, I was almost poisoned with the Stench.

Captain Burt was clearly something of a dandy, and may have found Edinburgh's habits more revolting than most. In fairness to him, however, it is reasonable to note what a very different sort of visitor had to say in his Journal in the year 1761. John Wesley, on a visit to Edinburgh, writes:

> The situation of the city is inexpressibly fine, and the main street so broad and finely paved . . . but how can it be suffered, that all manner of filth should still be thrown even into this street continually? How long shall the capital city of Scotland, yea, and the chief street of it, stink worse than a common sewer?[7]

This seems to sum up the ghastly picture of Scots hygiene in bygone centuries. Surely there has been progress in this field. Not for us the maggoty meat, grease-laden kitchens or flea-ridden bedrooms of our unfortunate ancestors. We may think with justifiable pleasure of our shining formica-topped kitchen units, our hygienically-wrapped food, our gleaming bathrooms. We may even pause for a moment to imagine what it must have been like for a mother to try to nurse a child with typhoid in a hovel (or even in a mansion) with no running water.

We face a very different kind of pollution today. The potential hazards of radioactive contamination are already well recognised. Likewise the use of artificial fertilisers, pesticides, fungicides; of antibiotics, both in animal husbandry and in food preservation; perhaps especially, the pollution of our waters by metallic residues, such as mercury, from industrial wastes: all of these pose serious problems for society today. Many medicals believe that susceptible persons are in fact already suffering from a wide range of reactions to such contaminants.

A quotation from John V Taylor's book *Enough is Enough* provides a salutary note on which to end this chapter:

> God forgive us if ever again we turn up supercilious white noses at the open drains of Asian and African cities, or snigger when we read again of that old cry from the upper windows of Edinburgh's mediaeval streets—Gardyloo!—which, as they learned from the euphemistic French of the Palace (beware of the water!) was the proper warning that the household slops were about to be flung out. For the world has had to wait until the arrival of scientific, technological man to see its rivers, seas and atmosphere not only treated as drains and sewers, but made to receive an ever-growing load of poisonous chemicals and gases, thermal and radioactive waste, harmful metallic substances, crude oil leaks, fertiliser and detergent run-off, inadequately treated sewage, and non-soluble containers.[8]

6

THE FOOD OF THE INDUSTRIAL POOR

What made it so bad?

> Take a fox and cutt the haire of and bruse the bones of itt . . . put
> them in a great Boylor, and lett boyll very Easyly for twenty-four
> Howrs. . . . Streane itt and put itt into the pot with speare mint and
> Rosemary sutherwood Harts Tungue Leverwirt strobery leavs time
> sweet margoram violett and leavs Balme jucy hop, of Each a good
> Handful. Take the Childe and put itt into a vessell to the Chin . . . and
> bath itt for half an Howr or longer as the Childe can indure, than take
> itt out and wipe itt and put itt into clean linen and lett go to bed.

This weird-sounding set of instructions, culled from the seventeenth-century Household Book of one of Scotland's great houses, may seem to us scarcely less strange when we discover that it was meant to constitute a cure of the times for rickets.

Rickets, that terrible disease of the bones which was to cause Scotland's slum-dwellers untold misery; which for many children would mean death; which condemned multitudes to go through life bow-legged and stunted; and which, through its effects upon pelvic bones, would mean agonisingly difficult childbirth for thousands of women. Sadly, while the above 'recipe' may sound quaintly amusing to modern ears, it has to be said that until the second and third decades of this present century, rickets and its causes were still very imperfectly understood. Even today many older city-dwellers carry its scars, reminding us of just one facet of the legacy of human suffering for which the rise to industrial prosperity must bear the blame.

Rickets and scurvy; smallpox and cholera; typhus and dysentery—these and many other ills were the lot of the industrial poor of the late eighteenth and the nineteenth centuries, as the Industrial Revolution got under way in Scotland, while villages swelled haphazardly to become towns, and small towns—with just as little thought for planning—grew into cities.

In previous chapters we have looked at some of the changes

which were taking place in eighteenth-century Scotland and affecting, in many areas, every aspect of social and agricultural life; in particular, how the improved farming techniques had made possible the production of locally-produced food of good quality. Had all things been equal, it seems clear that Scotland's then predominantly rural population—two thirds of whom are estimated to have lived in the Southern Uplands and Highlands—might have looked forward to a gradually improving lot. The reality, however, was vastly different. That watershed in the latter half of the eighteenth century, which marked the beginnings of so many rural changes, saw also the start of a coincidental movement which would result in Scotland's becoming a highly industrialised nation, and, while bringing undreamed-of wealth to some, would cause an infinitely greater number to live in extreme squalor. Ironically, one set of changes led indirectly to the other, for had there not arisen a food industry capable of feeding (after a fashion) large numbers of city dwellers, industrialisation on such a scale would have been out of the question.

Just when those changes began which would eventually mean a sharp divergence between rural and urban life—and not least in the matter of diet—is difficult to pin-point exactly: as in other fields, conditions varied widely from area to area. On this point William Ferguson points out:

> Historical perspective has been distorted by equating the eighteenth century with the Agrarian and Industrial Revolutions . . . in fact the post-Union period was marked by drifts and trends rather than by grandiose projects. This was very much the case with developments in agriculture, which were essentially piecemeal and localised, conforming to no one predetermined pattern.[1]

At some time dating from the early nineteenth century, however, it becomes impossible any longer to speak of 'the Scots diet': the differences between the wholesome, traditional rural fare and that of the cities becomes ever more apparent, with a corresponding difference in standards of health—and, most markedly, physique—of the people.

The contrast between the towns before and after the Industrial Revolution, too, could scarcely have been greater. About Glasgow, for example, Daniel Defoe could actually write in the early eighteenth century that it was 'the cleanest and beautifullest, and best built city in Britain, London excepted'.[2] It comes as something of a surprise, indeed, to find that in 1695 the Town Council of Glasgow had made it an offence for anyone to allow midden-heaps or fulyie (filth) to lie in the streets, or, in the following year, for anyone to throw out 'any excrement, dirt, or urine, or other filth, or water foul or clean', thus setting Glasgow ahead of the capital in this respect (although the actual enforcement of these orders seems to have taken a very long time).

Reading the entries for Glasgow in the *Statistical Account,* one cannot but observe the very absence of divergence between town and country in that final decade of the eighteenth century. The Glasgow report mentions, for example, that there exist ample markets for meat, fish, potatoes, butter and cheese. 'There is also a very commodious market', continues the writer, 'for the disposal of garden stuffs, the consumption of which is very considerably increased within these few years.'[3]

At that time, too, before the heavy industries had been generally established, the *Statistical Account*[4] casts light on the way in which the majority of industrial workers—then mainly employed in the textile trade—were then faring. The budget of a weaver's family in a Lanarkshire town, for example, is quoted in full. Here, the man and his wife both work as weavers, supporting three children under the age of five:

	£	s	d
Earnings at a medium per week	0	9	0
Earnings in a year	23	8	0
Expenses a-week			
3 pecks oatmeal, 2 pecks barley meal	0	3	8
Milk, salt, onions, potatoes	0	1	0
Butter, cheese, bacon, other meat	0	0	8
Soap, blue, starch, oil	0	0	6
Thread, thrum, worsted	0	0	1
	0	5	11
In a year	15	7	8
Excess	8	0	4

This type of worker, although labouring long hours in damp, ill-ventilated quarters, was at this very early stage of the industrial era at least managing to maintain a tolerable standard. His menu contains most of the basic necessities for health, although the common failing of the Scots diet of the times is again evident— paucity of vegetable foods. One cannot feel that a mere shilling to cover 'milk, salt, onions, potatoes' leaves room for very many potatoes, nor do we know whether kail or turnips would have been available if potatoes were not. Once again, therefore, it is likely that vitamin C would have been deficient at some time in the year.

However, this weaver's earnings set him well ahead of the agricultural workers of that time, the highest paid of whom were earning around £10 to £12 per annum.

As a comparison, the budget of an agricultural worker with a wife and four children under eight is reproduced in full below, from the *Statistical Account* for Moulin, in Perthshire:

Expenditure	£	s.	d.	Earnings	£	s.	d.
Food per week:				Man's earnings in 26 weeks			
3 pecks potatoes @ 4d.		1	0	spring & summer at 6s. per			
2 pecks oatmeal @ 11d.		1	10	week	7	16	0
2 pecks bere meal @ 7½d.		1	3				
Salt, *milk, *eggs, ale			6	4 weeks harvest			
		4	7	(plus victuals)	1	6	0
* milk 2d. per Scotch pint							
* eggs 2d. per dozen.				22 weeks, autumn & winter			
				at 3s. 6d.	3	17	0
Food per week		4	7	£	12	19	0
Food per annum	11	18	4				
				Wife's annual earnings			
(Deduct subsistence of man				from spinning	2	12	0
during harvest 1s. 10d. per				Total earnings £	15	11	0
week)							
This leaves	11	11	0				
House, rent, fuel etc.	2	1	6				
Clothing	3	8	9	*Deficiency* £	1	10	3
Total expenses £	17	1	3				

The writer of the report adds:

> Although there thus appears to be a deficiency of earnings, after the charges have been estimated in the most frugal, and even scanty manner, and no allowance made for casual expenses; yet it is certain, in this country, people who seem to have no livelihood but the fruits of their daily labour, do, by some means or other, bring up families, and even give their children such education as the nearest school affords.[5]

Moving back to the industrial scene, we find another contributor to the *Statistical Account* describing the diet of the child labourers in the cotton mills of New Lanark. Here, the proprietor was responsible for feeding and clothing his workers—keeping them extremely healthy by all accounts—as they must have required to be to sustain a working day which lasted from 6 a.m. till 7 p.m. with one-and-a-half hours for meals; after which they attended school until 9 p.m. Their diet was as follows:

> Oatmeal porridge or sowens with milk, as much as they can take. Barley broth for dinner made with good fresh beef every day, and as much beef is boiled as will allow 7 oz. English apiece each day to one

half of the children; the other half get cheese and bread after their broth, so that they dine alternately upon cheese and butchermeat, with barley bread and potatoes; and now and then in the proper season they get a dinner of herring and potatoes.[6]

A nutritional assessment of this diet reveals very good scores for practically all the nutrients, including those vital ones required for body-building. The children's physique must certainly have been significantly better than that of most of their contemporaries, for the proprietor, a known philanthropist, had ideas greatly in advance of his time.

Exceptional as these menus may have been, the other two examples quoted above show that generally the food of the urban population in the early years of the industrial era was substantially the same as that of the rural people. It is difficult to be certain to what extent 'bought bread' had begun to displace barley bannocks and oatcakes; it is likely, however, that this was happening more in the cities and in the smaller towns sufficiently near them. In the report for Lanark we read: 'Flour baked into bread comes all the way from Edinburgh and Glasgow, which greatly enhances the price of bread.'

The claim has been made that the first blasts of Falkirk's Carron Iron Works heralded the start of Scotland's Industrial Revolution. Certainly from around that time (1759) the race towards industrial expansion was on in earnest, and drastic changes in the whole of Scottish life were soon under way. Large factories began to take over from the old village-based trades, and thousands left the countryside to be swallowed up in the burgeoning heavy industries—coal-mining, heavy metal-working, ship-building—as well as in the giant jute, linen and cotton mills.

While judgements from a modern standpoint clearly have to be avoided, it is difficult to read of the conditions under which the poor of those days were forced to work without being appalled. In the bleachfields, children worked in heated chambers for between 14 and 18 hours a day; in the mines, women harnessed to bogeys dragged coal to the coal-face, their daily load estimated to be equivalent to carrying a hundredweight of coal from sea level to the summit of Ben Lomond. Colliers in general lived in a state of servitude to their employers. And all the time social conditions grew steadily worse as far too many people poured in, and widespread slums came into being in the Scottish cities.

This urban drift came from three directions—the Highlands, Ireland and the Lowlands. As early as between 1760 and 1783, an estimated 30,000 Highlanders, unable to make a living from the soil and thus destitute in times of scarcity, left their native lands. In 1782, for example, the pace was quickened when bad weather destroyed the crops and at the same time storms prevented fishing. 'Starving droves of Highlanders came south from impoverished crofts', writes Henry Graham, 'and, not too heartily, worked in the factories; ploughmen left the hills for the mills, and farmers were forced to raise their wages to keep workers in their service.'[7] In the *Statistical Account* for Callander we read:

> Where the people were most crowded, and the landlord had least money, there depopulation has made the widest strides; and the human race has been swept away as with a pestilence. The people in that large tract of country, from Kintyre to Ross, who are dispossessed of their farms, have no alternative but to cross the Atlantic, if they have spirit or wealth; or to travel southward, if they be poor. The villages of this place and other villages in similar situations, are filled with those naked and starving crowds of people, who are pouring down every term, for shelter or for bread.[8]

Thus began the trek south for the people of the Highlands, as it was to continue into the era of the Clearances and beyond. First, enclosure of the land and later the clamour in England for wool led to the ousting of many in favour of the more lucrative sheep-rearing; and those who had neither braved the rigours of an Atlantic crossing nor settled in the new coastal fishing communities ended up in the slums of the south. Nor did the two industries, fishing and kelp production, which had been expected to transform the Highland economy, bear out the optimism of the day; by 1815 things were as bad as ever.

From the north, too, came many more desperate folk in the wake of the disastrous famines of the mid-1840s, caused by the dreaded potato blight. In an earlier chapter we noted how dangerously potato-dependent Highland agriculture had by this time become; we saw too that certain lairds managed to tide their tenants over the disaster by providing work such as road-making.

This same famine swelled to a flood the stream of poor Irish immigrants who for a number of decades had been reaching south-west Scotland, thus greatly adding to the already desperate housing problem, and leading to a great deterioration of social conditions. By 1851 it was estimated that Irish immigrants constituted 7 per cent of the population of Scotland.

Agricultural advances in the Lowlands accounted for the third source of immigrants to the cities. It had become more profitable to incorporate numerous small holdings into large farms, with the result that many farm tenants found themselves with no alternative but to seek work in the towns. Small farmers and even some of the smaller gentry were swept away in the general depopulation.

It is impossible to consider diet in isolation from those other factors with which it is inextricably associated—housing, hygiene and health. Everywhere one turns, the picture speaks for itself— grim tenement buildings seething with people, to say nothing of rats and insects; one-room houses the norm, for large families and often a lodger as well; miners' houses with middens practically on the doorstep, and having one closet for the entire row. Writing of Glasgow in particular, Elizabeth Haldane says:

> There were no privies, and, as a considerable part of the rent of the houses was paid for by the produce of the dunghills, it would consequently be esteemed an invasion of the rights of property to remove them.[9]

Conditions were not improved by the fact that, due to the Window Tax, the houses of the poor had the tiniest of windows; in Edinburgh a whole row of houses was actually built without a single window in any of the bedrooms. With the best will in the world, one writer claimed, no woman could have kept her family clean in such surroundings. Nor was water easily available to aid her—not even for drinking, to say nothing of the luxury of washing. In the early nineteenth century, we find Glasgow with its population of some 80,000 dependent on about thirty wells on the main streets, where the people queued with their stoups for the privilege of receiving unfiltered water from the Clyde—into which more than two dozen small towns and villages poured their sewage. Not surprisingly, in 1804 an enterprising citizen had spring water piped into the centre of the city, serving the townsfolk at ½d. per stoup from his four-wheeled carts. Not until 1855 did an Act of Parliament ensure clean Loch Katrine water for Glasgow—water which, when it did eventually arrive, was not altogether welcomed by the populace on account of its lack of taste—and smell. The story of Edinburgh's water supply is strikingly similar.

Probably the peak of urban squalor was reached around the mid-nineteenth century. The Report on the Sanitary Conditions of the Labouring Population of Great Britain, published in 1842, noted that Glasgow was 'probably the filthiest and unhealthiest of all the British towns of this period'—and this not much more than a century after the accolade accorded by Daniel Defoe.

Around this time too the *New Statistical Account of Scotland*

was published—on the whole a much less diverting document than
the earlier one. Some of the contributors show concern over the
conditions in the industrial areas; others do not. Of Edinburgh's
poor, the writer says:

> The modern police regulations of the city are so complete as regards
> cleanliness, that the ancient reproach of the Scottish capital is now
> entirely removed. As respects the domestic cleanliness and comforts of
> the lower classes in the old town, however, much is still wanting—a
> more ample supply of water and public conveniences. Some idea of the
> crowded state of the poorer classes may be formed from the fact, that
> many of the large tenements of the old town contain from 100 to 150
> inmates, a whole family being crowded into an apartment not more
> than 12 or 14 feet square.[10]

The writer of the Dundee report, less sympathetic to the poor,
considered the practice of child labour to be attributable to the
parents' greed:

> It is extremely difficult to legislate betwixt master and servant in all
> cases; and it will be found on inquiry, that the wants of the parents,
> more than any desire on the part of their employers, have crowded our
> manufacturing establishments with very young children.

Of the conditions in the factories he writes:

> In health, every precaution is taken to guard against disease; and when
> any epidemic prevails, every attention is paid to such as are overtaken
> by it, and all due means used for their recovery.[11]

At roughly the same time, Glasgow's Chief Constable is on
record as having stated: 'There is everything that is wretched,
loathsome and pestilential.' The death-rate, from cholera and
smallpox in particular, was appallingly high: successive epidemics
ravaged the city in 1818, 1837, 1847, 1851, and—for the last
time—in 1867. Not surprisingly, drunkenness was rife.

The reformers had by then begun to move forward, however,
waging a campaign which can only be highlighted briefly in this
context. Unrest among labourers had resulted in the Reform Bill
(1832), while the Chartist Movement of the 1840s, and the institu-
tion of Trade Unions, each played a powerful part. The Trade
Union Act of 1871 was an important step forward. Such amenities
as Friendly Societies added their benefits, and efforts were made
gradually to provide recreation grounds and open spaces for adults
and children.

Very importantly, in the field of health and hygiene, too, reforms began to follow one another in quick succession: Glasgow's first Medical Officer of Health in 1863; the Sanitary Office in 1864; the first Fever Hospital in 1865; the Scottish Public Health Act in 1867. Scotland's medical men, many of them by that time highly skilled and famous, spear-headed improvements in hospital conditions, while by the end of the century the old nursing standards were steadily being replaced by those laid down by Florence Nightingale.

Returning to consider the diet of the industrial poor, we find throughout the nineteenth century a pernicious deterioration of the traditional Scots diet. It is helpful here to look back briefly to the budget of the weaving family (which was quoted in full in the *Statistical Account*), using their diet as a barometer of change. In that last decade of the eighteenth century, we may recall, they were managing to make ends meet, with a credit balance of £8 per annum, the items of their food bill comprising predominantly oatmeal and barley meal, as well as potatoes and small amounts of milk, butter, cheese, bacon, onions and salt. By the mid-nineteenth century, however, most weavers were in dire straits. The advent of power looms had brought unemployment and poverty to the hand-loom weavers, and discontent was rife. Writing of the bread riots in the year 1848, Elizabeth Haldane writes:

> It was just after the potato famine and potatoes were still dear, and it was before the repeal of the Corn Laws had taken effect. The power-looms were in full swing, and there was great unemployment and depression amongst weavers.[12]

In Glasgow, this distress led to looting and general disorder, ending with the reading of the Riot Act. In Paisley alone, it was estimated that during the 'hungry forties' 10,000 men were unemployed. It is likely that our weaving family along with many others were by this time facing severe privation resulting in malnutrition. Workers in the heavy industries at that time should have been faring better, for they had steady employment, but the devastating potato famines of the mid-1840s must have hit not only the Irish and the Highlanders but all the poor of the day.

What were those dietary changes which led to a steady downward spiral in Scotland from the start of the nineteenth century onwards? First, there was the gradual replacement of oatmeal and barley meal by 'bought bread'. Bread, which had started as a nourishing wholemeal, scarcely less valuable than oatmeal itself, finally became virtually white after the introduction around 1870 of steel roller mills; at this time too, harmful bleaching agents were being added to flour. The only beneficiaries of the public demand for white bread were the millers, who were able to make a healthy profit from selling the bran as cattle fodder; for the townsfolk there must have been a considerable nutritional deterioration.

The year 1870 saw not only the loss of the more nutritious loaf but also of the butter to spread on it, for in that year the new food called margarine was first introduced in France as an inferior suet-based product: the later process of hardening vegetable oils by hydrogenation produced a cheap margarine which did not, as modern legislation requires, contain the important vitamins A and D.

While the devaluation of bread and butter, the staples of the poor, constitutes the main retrograde step in diet, there were others of lesser importance as well. We noted earlier how tea had gradually come to replace the more nourishing ale. There was, too, the gradual change from black treacle to syrup: although this might seem hardly significant, in fact 3 oz of treacle (a likely amount when it is remembered that bread was the main food) would provide about three-quarters of the calcium requirement of an adult, and one-quarter of the iron. Hand-in-hand with the liking for syrup went a demand for poor-quality jams made from vegetable pulp, and for other sweet, inexpensive products. Consumption of sugar and its products grew out of all proportion, with a consequent lowering of nutritional status.

This altogether unsatisfactory health situation was compounded by the failure to produce and distribute sufficient food for the needs of the city populations. Perhaps most deficient of all was the supply of milk, most vital of all foods for children. Until the advent of pasteurisation, around 1890, milk was not only unhygienic but also—until chemists exposed the practice—frequently watered-down. Since it was customary to bring cows to the towns after they had calved and to keep them there in far from clean conditions, the milk, either through bovine disease to start with or from later contamination, reached the people in a potentially dangerous state. During the course of the nineteenth century, condensed milk gained in popularity, but in this case too the popular taste for sweet foods meant that the sweetened variety made from skimmed milk—a by-product of the butter factories—was preferred, the valuable fat content of the milk thus being lost to the consumers. It was during the nineteenth century, however, that a new way of using milk did become popular: milk puddings using cereals began to be part of the daily menu.

Meat and its products played but a small part in the diet of the industrial poor—and just as well perhaps, since by all accounts the 'fresh' meat which was available was frequently of poor quality or actually putrefied. Knowledge of food preservation, although so urgently needed, had been confined almost exclusively to the ancient traditional methods of salting meat and smoking fish. Around 1860, however, canned meat arrived on the market, and this product, coming mainly from Chicago, gradually won favour with the Scots. Apart from this, an occasional meal of bacon or cheese was the most likely addition to the predominantly starchy diet of the poor.

The *New Statistical Account* makes it clear nevertheless that some enterprising industrialists in Scotland had become interested in the canning of food earlier in the century. In the account for Leith, for example, we read of an interesting development in food technology:

> An establishment for the preservation of all kinds of fresh meat and vegetables for naval stores &c. was commenced in 1838. The principle of this manufactory consists in cooking and enclosing in airtight tin cases all sorts of soups, flesh and fish, and vegetable substances, and carefully excluding all contact with atmospheric air. In this way the various meats keep in all climates for many years, and afford a most convenient supply of provisions for travellers and voyagers. Milk, cream, gravies and jellies for invalids are also included in these ingenious processes.[13]

We do know that the need to provision ships for polar exploration gave added impetus to the search for methods of food preservation; indeed, caches of tinned foods have been recovered from the Arctic in this present century. As might be expected, there were not nearly enough to meet the demand. The report continues: 'The demand for these articles, both for home and foreign consumpt, is always more than even this extensive establishment can well accomplish.' All the same, Scotland was at last on the way to discovering new ways of feeding her burgeoning urban population.

Consumption of vegetables and fruit was extremely low, such as did reach the town markets being, not surprisingly, often far from fresh. Fruit in particular was expensive and generally beyond the reach of the poor. It should be remembered that for those living near the markets there may well have been an occasional Saturday night bargain to be had; the account quoted above of the Leith manufacturers of canned goods mentions, too, the kind of spin-off which might have come the way of the poor and eased their lot even a little: 'Some of the rejected oily matters of the cooking process are sold for greasing machinery; and other substances are purchased at a moderate price by the poor in the neighbourhood.'

In attempting to sum up the diet of the industrial poor of the nineteenth century, one would have to say that it was, on the whole, nutritionally inadequate, unhygienic and of poor quality. As we saw in Chapter 5, too, much of the food was subject to adulteration. But against this gloomy background should be set three extra food sources which were capable of making significant contributions to the diet of many people, even indeed of transforming it altogether. There were available, at least for some of the people some of the time, potatoes, buttermilk, and fresh foods from sea and countryside.

As we saw in Chapter 2, potatoes played a fundamental part in the Scottish economy from about the 1770s onwards, especially in the Highlands and Islands and among the poorer Lowland folk. Grown at first around the villages and small towns for the use of the inhabitants only, they later began to be produced commercially around the cities (making use, it may be added, of the liberal supplies of dung so readily available) as part of a new attempt in Scotland to grow enough food for her expanding urban population. With the growth of railways it became possible to transport potatoes to the city markets from further afield, a fact which accounts for Ayrshire's rise to potato-growing fame. Thus the increasing demands of an under-fed, under-paid population for a cheap but filling food had begun at least partially to be fulfilled. The contribution made by this one root vegetable to the otherwise almost vegetable-free diet of the city poor is one which can hardly be emphasised too strongly.

The second extenuating factor was the availability of buttermilk, in some quarters at least. For any city-dweller who had regular access to this excellent food the outlook so far as nutrition was concerned was without doubt greatly improved. The practice of taking soor-dook (buttermilk) into the cities from farms on the outskirts is still commemorated in such folk-songs as the one entitled, 'Ridin' doon tae Glesca wi' ma soor milk cairt'.

Lastly, there were the wares of the street vendors, who formed a colourful part of the urban scene during the nineteenth century. And a surprisingly wide range of foods they offered to those with money to buy. 'Wha'll buy neeps?' was the cry of the turnip-sellers, generally two girls carrying a clothes-basket between them. Then there were the barrows selling hot potatoes, surely a welcome sight in pre-chip days. In freezing weather, they catered not only for the poor, but were even bought by gentlemen for their ladies to hold

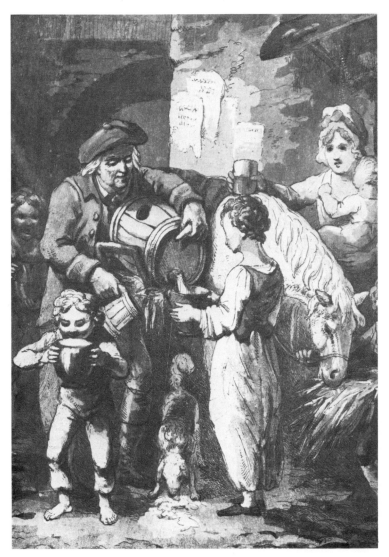

11 'Sour Milk', *Cries of Edinburgh*; aquatint by Robert Scott after John Burnett, *c.* 1805. *Source* National Galleries of Scotland, Edinburgh.

inside their muffs as hand-warmers. Most kenspeckle of all were the fishwives. The customary dialogue between customer and seller has been recorded thus: 'Whit price haddies the day, Janet?' To which the reply was: 'Haddies is men's lives the day, Mem.' Herrings sold for 2*d*. the dozen. There were also caller ou (fresh oysters), garvies (sprats), rock partons (crabs), and whelks, and even bunches of dulse and tangle from the sea-shore. Fruits too were sold on the streets in season—cherries, pears, apples, oranges, grossets (gooseberries), strawberries, raspberries. And the list of vegetables, besides potatoes and turnips, included leeks, radishes, cress, peas and beans. Even various cuts of cheeses could sometimes be bought.

It will be evident that this wide range of optional extras could change the nutritional picture quite considerably. In attempting to offer any assessment of the diet of the nineteenth century industrial population, one is hampered by lack of exact knowledge of the amounts available, even more than in the case of the rural labourers whose diet we looked at earlier. Suppose, however, that we take the *basic* diet per day of a male industrial worker in one of the Scottish cities as being

white bread	10 oz
sugar	3 oz
margarine	2 oz
syrup or jam	2 oz
condensed milk (skimmed) in tea	2 oz

It needs no complicated calculation to reveal a diet composed predominantly of carbohydrate, seriously lacking in every one of the essential minerals and vitamins. The bread lacked the valuable germ and bran; the margarine was not vitamin-enriched. Even the energy content is low for a hard-working man: the chances that the women and children would fare better are slim indeed. No wonder that this kind of food gave rise to a stunted population, suffering from every possible deficiency ranging from anaemia all the way through to the two scourges of the day—scurvy and rickets. In addition, it need hardly be said that they were an easy prey to every kind of infectious disease for which the unhygienic background too easily made way.

Suppose, however, that we now add to the above list a quantity of potatoes—say ¾ lb—which is a quite likely amount at some times of the year at least: this alone would make a considerable difference, enhancing not only the energy value but supplying significant amounts of mineral elements and, especially, B vitamins

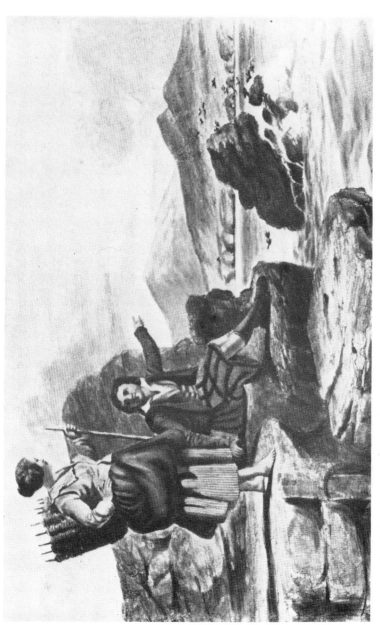

12 Gathering dulse. From McIan, *Highlanders at Home* 105. *Source* National Museum of Antiquities of Scotland, C2803.

and vitamin C. Of this last, it may be added that no matter how badly cooked the potatoes might have been from our modern viewpoint, they should have supplied more than enough to keep scurvy at bay.

Suppose, finally, that we add to this list a selection of those other foods from sea and countryside which could be bought on the streets—by those enjoying steady employment, presumably, or by the thrifty and weel-daein'. Buttermilk or cheese would add protein and calcium, so vital for the growth of children's bones, as well as the scarce vitamins of the B group; herrings would bring their contribution of protein and fat, along with the essential minerals and the vitamins A and D; vegetables and fruits in their seasons would enhance the mineral and vitamin content of the diet. It is more than likely too that many people had retained the healthy Scots habit of having porridge or brose once a day or more, or had remained faithful to oatcakes in preference to bread, something which would have paid high dividends as regards health. Much would have depended upon the availability of cooking facilities, however, and these were clearly of the most primitive in the worst of the slums. Those families who managed to achieve a menu which included such items as barley broth, oatmeal, butter, treacle, potatoes, turnips, milk (whether fresh, condensed, or buttermilk), with occasional meals of meat, fish or cheese, with extra vegetables and fruit in season, certainly had the basis of a perfectly adequate diet.

Looking at the Scotland of the era of the Industrial Revolution gives rise to some mixed impressions. On the one hand we see great achievement, as a country once proverbial for its poverty rises to fame—not simply as a rich industrial nation, but also for its excellence in agriculture. We read too of the outstanding contribution of brilliant Scots in the realms of literature, philosophy, engineering, medicine, law, natural history. Nor was literacy confined to the professional classes: all over the country we find poor people struggling to educate their children, and libraries and literary societies flourishing.

The other side of the coin need hardly be stressed. Scotland's gains included not only agricultural advances and industrial wealth but also slums and slag-heaps, poverty and ugliness; her losses in terms of rural traditions and culture would be difficult to estimate.

The social historian, Elizabeth Haldane, who made a detailed study of the period, sums up her impressions thus:

The new industries that arose brought many advantages. They brought wealth to the country and enabled a large number of people who had been living in poverty to earn good wages and enjoy greater comfort. The evil was that the employers considered that once they had created these industries their work was done; they had made no provision for the influx of men, women and children who crowded into the cities, nor did they see that this was a duty. Public authorities also disclaimed responsibility, as ratepayers emphatically did, and thus the consequences were disastrous.[14]

7

THE EARLY TWENTIETH CENTURY

Were the Scots now better fed?

In the year 1901, Edwin Muir, after a boyhood spent in Orkney, moved with his family to Glasgow. In his book *Scottish Journey* he describes the impact of this experience:

> When I arrived in Glasgow straight from Orkney, I had no self-protective apparatus for selecting my impressions, and was stunned by a succession of sights which I frantically strove not to see. . . . The slums not only penetrate the lives of all classes in Glasgow, but also send out a dirty wash into the neatest and remotest suburbs and even the surrounding countryside, so that it is possible for one to feel that the whole soil for miles around is polluted.[1]

It was not only the city itself that Muir found depressing. Of industrial Lanarkshire he writes:

> The forlorn villages, looked like dismembered parts of towns hacked off, and with the raw edges nakedly exposed. The towns themselves, on the other hand, were like villages on a nightmare scale, which after endless building had never managed to produce anything like a street, and had no centre of any kind. . . . Round those bloated and scabbed villages there are ranges of slag-heaps, miniature mountain ranges.

In trying to re-create and understand the past, we have seen repeatedly how fascinating light can be shed by the works of impressionable, sensitive writers. Clearly, however, we have to be carefully objective in our interpretation and use of such insights. In this instance, Muir's Orkney boyhood must surely have predisposed him to find the sudden transportation to the squalor of the industrial belt more than ordinarily overwhelming. But even the most cursory look at the social conditions of the urban Scots of the early twentieth century—even a look at a photograph of that era—conveys a strong impression of bleakness, drabness and poverty.

It would be quite wrong to suggest, however, that things had not changed, and changed fairly radically, since the days of the potato famines of the 1840s, when starving Irish and Highland folk had thronged to the cities in search of work and food. Gone, certainly, were the dunghills, the water queues, the dreaded visitations of the worst of the plagues. And although it might well be claimed that the changes were of degree only, it could also justifiably be claimed that had the people of the mid nineteenth century been able to see their descendants of the early twentieth century, they would have thought them privileged indeed.

Housing, nevertheless, was still an immense problem. While the census of 1861 had revealed that 226,723 families—some one-third of Scotland's entire population—were living in 'houses' of one room, as late as 1918 it was estimated that nearly half of the population still lived in grossly over-crowded conditions. City tenements still suffered from glaring faults—inadequate lighting and ventilation; communal stairhead privies; damp, malodorous basements. Nor were these faults confined to city dwellings—the numerous miners' rows of the smaller industrial towns and villages manifestly exhibited some of the worst features.

But what of the people's diet? We last looked at the food of Scotland's industrial poor during the latter half of the nineteenth century, when industrialisation was proceeding apace. How, if at all, had it improved since then? On the whole there does seem to have been some improvement, although as always no simple overall answer is possible. Even if there existed, for reference, neatly tabulated menus and accounts of food expenditure for any given period, a detailed picture might be slow to emerge. Instead, it is a question of varying conditions in different parts of the country, even within the same city; of differences between the employed and the unemployed, the thrifty and the prodigal. Sometimes it is necessary to use conjecture rather than solid fact.

The Englishman's Food,[2] Drummond and Wilbraham's classic review of the diet in England through the centuries, contains a depressing reference to the general state of nutrition during this era: 'It is no exaggeration to say that the opening of the 20th century saw malnutrition more rife in England than it had been since the great dearths of mediaeval times.' And sadly, what was true south of the Border is likely to have been at least equally true of industrial Scotland. The following list of foods is quoted directly from *The Englishman's Food* as a typical 'poverty diet' of the time:

| | *Per day* | | |
Foods	Weight	Protein (g)	Kcalories
Bread	1½ lb	52.8	1,656
Sausages	2 oz	7.8	162
Potatoes	4 oz	1.6	92
Banana (one)	3 oz	1.0	66
Condensed milk	1 oz	2.8	76
Cocoa	1 oz	5.8	128
Jam	2 oz	—	148
Sugar	2 oz	—	224
Margarine	2 oz	—	452
		71.8	3,004

While these foods would have provided just enough energy, in other respects—notably the vital mineral and vitamin constituents—the diet is seriously deficient. Interestingly, though, the protein content, which earlier experts would have thought inadequate, would today be regarded as sufficient: of its approximate 70 g, most is contributed by bread which—refined or not—provides a surprising amount.

It has often been pointed out that the diet cannot properly be studied in isolation from social conditions. Here the connection is self-evident. Not only did the poor eat a diet of this kind because they could afford no other: the extremely basic cooking facilities available to most of them also dictated the enormous demand for bread, and led too to the choice of the frying-pan as a cooking utensil—a choice which is still in many areas evident today. In addition, there was an almost total ignorance of food values—shared to some extent by the medical profession—food being on the whole regarded as something to allay hunger.

The detrimental consequences of such a diet are not far to seek. Anaemia through lack of iron and other blood-forming nutrients; scurvy always a possibility, especially in winter and spring, from lack of vegetables and fruit; gross dental decay from the high sugar content; stunting of growth because of the serious lack of vitamin and mineral growth factors. And as in previous centuries, rickets, that most obvious of all the deficiency diseases of the slums, continued relentlessly to attack countless children. If to all these hazards are added the poor standards of housing and of working conditions, the generally unsatisfactory physique of the industrial population was only to be expected.

Records of births and deaths have always provided illuminating insights into the health of a people. Of these statistics—kept from the year 1855 onwards in Scotland by the Registrar-General—the most telling are those for infant mortality: the close correlation between food and health during the first year of life has long been recognised. In 1855, no fewer than 125 infants per 1,000 failed to survive their first year. By the turn of the century the figure had actually risen slightly, but it declined thereafter to reach around 70 in the 1930s (and around 20 in the 1970s).

Something else which has been recognised for a long time is that the stature of a people can be a strong indication of its nutritional status. As early as 1883, for example, it was recorded that 13-year-old schoolboys from a poor industrial area were on average 5.8 inches shorter than their contemporaries from a professional background. But it was at the time of the South African War (1899–1902) that the generally poor physique—not just in Scotland but in the UK as a whole—really came to light and began to cause great concern. The Army authorities were having difficulty in finding sufficient recruits of a suitable standard, the rejection rate in certain areas being as high as 50 per cent.

The year 1906 is notable in the history of nutrition for two important forward steps. The first is the start of an official school feeding programme. Following the distressing disclosures by the Army recruiting drives of widespread malnutrition and sub-standard physique among young people, it was realised that those charitable schemes by which some food was supplied to some needy children were quite inadequate, and a report followed which led to the Education Act (Provision of Meals) 1906. Although far removed from the streamlined School Meals Service which we tend nowadays to take for granted, this did ensure some food—on schooldays—for the most deprived children. Under the provisions of this Act local authorities continued to supply meals for school-children up to the time of the First World War—when, sadly, there was a pronounced decline, in the interests of economy. At the time under-nutrition was by no means confined to the children of the poor; feeding standards in the private boarding schools were generally unsatisfactory, and were to remain so for many years to come.

The year 1906 is memorable, too, for a significant happening of a totally different kind. In that year a Cambridge scientist made the following statement (his research, however, having been shared with others before): 'No animal can live on a mixture of proteins, carbohydrates, and fats; and even when the necessary inorganic material is carefully supplied, the animal still cannot flourish.'[3] On

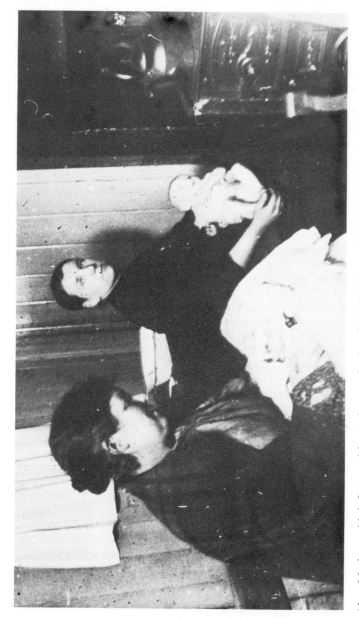

13　Mothers with infants waiting to be examined at the Milk Depot, 106 Maitland Street, Glasgow, *c.* 1911. *Source* Strathclyde Regional Archives.

the face of it, perhaps, not a very earth-shattering statement—not, that is, unless one realises that until then scientists had believed animals could survive on just these very nutrients. The food chemists around the turn of the century had, in fact, believed their understanding of nutrition to be virtually complete. They had investigated not only the combustion of food within the human body, but also the role of the proteins, starches, sugars and fats, not to mention several mineral elements. Their dismay, therefore, at finding that young animals fed on a highly purified mixture of these nutrients failed to thrive and finally declined and died, can well be imagined. The baffling discovery that only the addition of small amounts of natural foods (such as milk) ensured the survival of the animals, sparked off the most exciting chapter in the whole history of nutrition, one which was to last until around the mid-century. It was the search for those most elusive of all food factors, the vitamins—a search which unfortunately cannot be pursued in this particular study—which was to have, in the end, far-reaching consequences for the Scottish diet.

Fortunately these two steps forward—one in public health and the other in the laboratory—are not the only items on the credit side in the food situation in Scotland early in this century. Not only did the majority of working folk by now have at least enough food to live on—more than could have been said of preceding genera-tions—but for some of them at least, principally those in better-paid jobs or with small families, rising living conditions had brought far more articles of diet within reach, so that by the first decade of the century the diet of many could well have been reaching quite acceptable standards. From the 1870s onwards, for example, the consumption of wheat had been falling and that of meat rising—always a feature of increasing affluence—the meat being largely canned, imported first from Australia and the USA, and later from South America. Not only were eggs and cheese more generally in use, and the hygiene of the milk supply much improved after the adoption of pasteurisation in the 1890s; there was also beginning to emerge in the cities and some of the towns that celebrated food partnership which would one day characterise the British diet, fish and chips. Whatever our attitude to these foods, whether we are among those who deride them or the many more who enjoy them, we should on no account fail to recognise their immense contribution to the diet of Scotland's urban poor, the fish providing excellent body-building material, the chips becoming for very many the only really reliable source of vitamin C.

The 'poverty diet' already quoted, with its great preponderance

of bread, refers specifically to England. In Scotland, a large proportion of families continued to use the much superior oatmeal,
although their numbers did decline as the years went on. As we saw
in an earlier chapter, too, two other cheap foods, treacle and
cocoa, added much of value (particularly iron) to the daily diet.
The consumption of vegetables and fruit, although slightly higher
than in the previous century, continued to be unacceptably low.

This roughly sums up the position at the outbreak of the First
World War in 1914. One of the first consequences of this was,
predictably, a sharp rise in food prices, which was estimated by
halfway through the war as 65 per cent. The exception was sugar:
its price rose by an unprecedented 163 per cent. Bread—designated
'Government bread' from the end of 1916—was at first simply a
higher-extraction and thus more nutritious loaf, but later received
such additions as bean and potato flour.

Of considerable interest is the series of guides to economical
eating published by the National Food Economy League. 'Housekeeping on Twenty-five Shillings a week, for a Family of Five' took
care of the lower orders, while for the others there was, for
example, 'Patriotic Food Economy for the Well-to-do'. Making
liberal use of cheap but nourishing foods like beans, lentils, green
and root vegetables, and wholegrain cereals, they had a great deal
to commend them, and if carefully followed could certainly have
led to an improvement in health. But the chief difficulty was that as
the war dragged on it was becoming harder and harder for the
housewife to obtain sufficient food of any kind. In December 1915
The Times reported:

> The food queues continue to grow. Outside the dairy shops of certain
> multiple firms in some parts of London, women begin to line up for
> margarine as early as 5 o'clock on Saturday morning, some with
> infants in their arms.

Queues for potatoes, too, were a common sight. *The Times* also
reported tea, sugar, butter, margarine, lard, dripping, milk, rice,
currants, raisins, wines and spirits all in short supply. In 1918,
rationing (of meat, tea, butter) was finally introduced. That in
some quarters there was serious malnutrition is more than likely;
some have claimed that there was a sharp increase in the incidence
of scurvy, although this would be hard to prove. Certainly many
have seen the devastating effects of the great influenza epidemic,
which arrived in June 1918, as being due at least in part to the
generally under-nourished state of the nation.

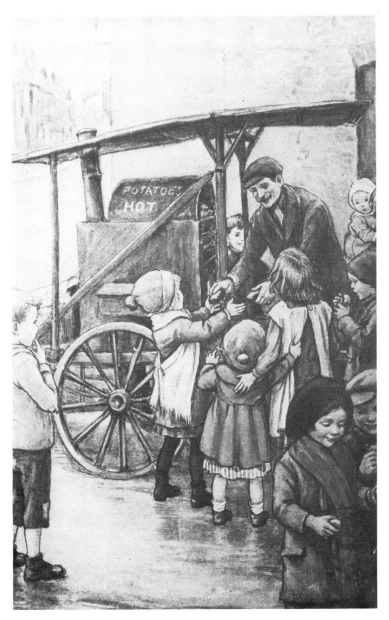

14   Hot Potatoes. From *Jolly Pictures*. (Blackie & Sons, Glasgow)

The period of widespread industrial unrest which followed the war has left us one interesting piece of information on the diet of workers of that era, although again, admittedly, referring specifically to South of the Border. The dockers—labouring at the time under most unsatisfactory conditions—having put forward a claim for a wage of sixteen shillings a day, a professor at London University had, at the request of the employers, drawn up a minimum weekly budget for a man, his wife and three young children.[4] Allowing £2 (out of a total of £3.13s. 6d.) for food, it consisted of the following amounts:

Meat	6 lb	Rice	2 lb
Bacon	1 lb	Sugar	2½ lb
Sausages (or fish)	2 lb	Jam	2½ lb
Cheese	11½ oz	Biscuits	12 oz
Milk	8 pints	Lard or suet	1 lb
Margarine	2 lb	Tea	10 oz
Bread	21 lb	Cocoa	4 oz
Flour	7 lb	Fruit	tenpence-worth
Oatmeal		Peas	
(or other cereal)	1 lb	Carrots	one shilling's
		Cabbage	worth
		Potatoes	14 lb

In court, a spirited argument arose between the professor (for the employers) and socialist politician Ernest Bevin (for the dockers). The latter, contesting that the professor's budget was totally inadequate for a family of five, took the trouble to buy, cook and bring to court the exact amounts of food specified, and laid them out as exhibits. Clearly his main target was the meat portion of the diet: the bacon, for example, he divided up into five tiny servings for each day to show how derisory they were. Today, interestingly, our criticisms are quite different: we would consider bacon for breakfast unnecessary and 6 lb of meat plus 2 lb of sausages more than adequate, but would deplore instead the lack of milk, eggs, cheese, whole cereals, vegetables and fruit. Thus do nutritional mores change!

This diet—based on the actual food of a railway porter's family in 1914—can hardly be classed as a 'poverty diet'. Perhaps what it illustrated most clearly is the vast improvement which had, generally speaking, taken place in the food of the poorer section of England's population by around 1920. All the same, it is questionable whether many working families would have been able to spend as much as £2 weekly on food, in view of the average earnings at the time. (For those who like to hear the end of a story—the dockers were awarded their sixteen shillings a day.)

The above budget catered, clearly, for the specific needs and tastes of English labourers. How were the Scots faring by 1920? Although details of food consumption are not readily available, a number of family dietary studies were carried out, chiefly in Glasgow and Edinburgh, between 1900 and the early 1920s. Outstanding among these is a comprehensive Report by the Medical Research Council (MRC Report No. 101), published in 1925 but covering the years from 1919 onwards, and embodying studies among Scots labouring families, principally in Glasgow, Edinburgh and Dundee, but also including some in mining and agricultural areas.[5] Led by two professors, the researchers undertook a special study of the nutrition and health of children—something not previously attempted—and in particular set out to demonstrate decisive links between child nutrition and family income. It was, for the time, an immense task. The authors wrote:

> The difficulties of understanding the relationship of nutrition and growth to food supply are very great. Do the country children eat greater amounts because they are bigger and more active, or are they bigger and more active because they eat more?

Information was painstakingly collected—on weekly income and rent, food expenditure, number of persons, number of rooms, airspace per person; and, naturally, the children were weighed and measured. Yet, strangely, the researchers failed in their main quest, that of establishing clear links between family income and child nutrition. Why was this? Probably because, as was normal practice at the time, they concentrated on assessing protein and fat and, above all, energy (calorie) intakes, and finding these generally adequate, missed the serious lack of vitamin and mineral constituents. Thus they failed to pinpoint the glaring faults of a diet which was responsible for the slum child's stunted growth and, especially, rickets. Just as researchers of an earlier day had tended to attribute most of the ills of the poor to ignorance, alcoholism, overcrowding and poor sanitation, so in this Report the stunted growth was seen as resulting from 'racial influences', exacerbated by overcrowding and lack of fresh air and sunlight. Although they were obviously moving towards understanding, the full realisation of the vital role of diet had to wait one decade more.

The First World War is regarded as a watershed in the economic history of Scotland. At the time of this Report, for example, she was already in the grip of depression: loss of foreign markets, coupled with more complex factors, were causing contraction in exports, so that for some time after the General Strike in 1926, Scottish exports fell behind those of the UK as a whole. Unemployment was rife, and although the heavy industries (and thus the Clyde area in the west) suffered most, industries such as linen and jute in the east were also contracting, a fact which is reflected in that part of the Report devoted to Dundee families in whom the bread-winner was unemployed.

The Report provides many interesting insights quite apart from nutrition. It paints a clear, often painfully clear, picture of social conditions in Scotland in those years following the First World War. We read in some detail of conditions in the city slums; of pale, sickly children; of some mothers who had simply abandoned the unequal struggle against poverty and dirt, and of yet others who somehow managed to maintain an amazingly high standard in the face of both. There are studies of 'good working-class families' with reasonable living conditions and wholesome food, compared with others in whom the bread-winner is unemployed and where a hand-to-mouth existence is the norm, where life is possible only through continual borrowing from neighbours and credit from shops, together with a pittance from the Labour Bureau and Parish Relief. 'These families', states the Report, 'did very little cooking. The main diet consisted of bread and margarine; in fact most of the pots and pans had been pawned.'

There are, too, comparisons between the mothers' performances in domestic management, one of the criteria being the number of calories they managed to purchase for one penny. In the mining districts, mothers were judged to maintain far higher standards of cleanliness than their city counterparts, although it is suggested that some seemed more intent on keeping their houses polished than on feeding their children. Despite their apparent lack of any tradition of preparing a midday meal for their children (who simply cut themselves a 'piece') the standard of child health was rated far higher than in the cities.

Interesting differences, too, emerge between Glasgow and Dundee. Despite the generally poor housing prevalent in the latter, the health of the children is considered superior, and strikingly so in one important aspect—the incidence of rickets. Mothers in Dundee, the Report explains, were aware to a quite surprising extent of their children's need for open air and sunshine. They not only made all possible use of outside stairs and balconies, and of all available parks; they also endeavoured whenever possible to reach open countryside—a much more accessible amenity generally than in Glasgow. The Report concludes:

> Rickets is much more prevalent and more severe in Glasgow than in Dundee. It is now recognised that the condition is associated with a deficiency of sunshine and fresh air. . . . Dundee enjoys this to a much greater extent than does Glasgow. In the latter city it is the careful mothers alone who can secure for their children a modicum of these, and who may succeed in rearing them free of rickets.

This last statement is of especial interest. By the year in which the Report was published (1925), the complex, baffling problem of the causation of rickets, and in particular the preventive role of sunshine, had just been more or less disentangled. Before we reach that point, however, it is necessary to look backwards.

Rickets, ably described by two English physicians as early as the mid seventeenth century, had doubtless been known in the sunless lands of Northern Europe from early times. In that century it was being studied extensively both in Britain and in Europe, and the simple cure—which indeed has never been bettered—was known to at least a few. Much later, in a brilliant account of the disease, an eighteenth century French physician was able to write: 'Cod liver oil is the well-known and perfect cure for rickets.' Alas, it was not well-known to all; although in 1782 an English doctor described the 'loathsomeness' of the oil, produced by 'heaping together the livers of the fish, from which, by gentle putrefaction, the oil flows very plentifully'. Evidence exists that the cure was known to Northern European peasants for many centuries, and that fish liver oils were also used by Hebridean people—sometimes swallowed, sometimes rubbed on—although chiefly as a treatment for rheumatism and tuberculosis. The use of seal oil for medicinal purposes is, however, still well remembered today by elderly people from the Western Isles.

In looking at the effects of the Industrial Revolution in the last chapter, we touched briefly on the subject of rickets, noting how increasing industrialisation had caused a colossal increase in its incidence in all the cities of Britain. Not surprisingly, in Scotland it became known as 'the Glasgow disease'. The cause, as is now well known, was two-fold. First, the diet was deficient in both calcium and vitamin D. For the proper hardening of bone, calcium salts are required, while vitamin D has a vital function in depositing them. In a deficiency, therefore, normal bone formation is impossible and the weight-bearing parts of the skeleton suffer, resulting in various deformities—of legs, pelvis, spine—some of which, indeed, are still visible in elderly city-dwellers today. But vitamin D is, of course, also formed in the body by the action of sunlight. This source, too, was denied to the unfortunate children of the slums, since the high tenements and the thick pall of industrial smoke effectively shut it out.

The story of rickets makes some of the saddest reading in the whole of Scotland's social history. If ever there was a disease of sheer deprivation, this surely was it. For us today, accustomed as we are to seeing our children grow up strong and straight-limbed, it requires a distinct effort of imagination to picture the thousands of miserable children with every kind of bone deformity—bow-legged, knock-kneed, pigeon-chested—unable to enjoy the delights of normal active childhood, and a prey to infection at the same time. Perhaps in retrospect the saddest aspect of all is that a simple and cheap treatment was available, so cheap that even the poorest just might have been able to procure it. But rickets is a classic example of a complex and baffling disease for which new treatments were constantly being tried, while the careful research of previous centuries was forgotten.

Up to the year 1919, the year which saw the start of the Medical Research Council's Report on child health in Scotland, an amazing amount of confusion existed about rickets. There were three principal theories—first, that it was caused by an infective agent; second, that it was due to a vitamin deficiency (although this school was then confusing this with another fat-soluble factor, later identified as vitamin A); the third, that it had its origin in lack of exercise, fresh air and sunlight. Researchers holding this last view, notably the Glasgow School, were clearly groping towards recognition of the involvement of sunshine in their measurements, for example of the airspace available to each child.

If we are tempted to feel impatient with the seeming blindness of the medical men of the day, it is as well to imagine how truly baffling the problem was. How tempting to attribute to an infection (especially in the wake of Pasteur's discoveries) a disorder affecting whole families; how remote, on the other hand, the connection between a bone disease and sunshine. Especially hard for us to understand, perhaps, is the difficulty caused by the concept of a disease of deficiency. In former times, diseases were believed to be *caused by* some agent—poison, cold, damp, alcoholism—but, as we saw in the case of scurvy earlier, the idea that they could actually have their origins in any *lack* was extremely slow of acceptance.

In 1919, however, the study of rickets was at last about to take a significant step forward. In that year a British medical team went to Vienna to study the disease under the appalling conditions of post-war famine then prevailing in that city. By the time their final report was published (1923), much of the perplexity had been dispelled. They had demonstrated that the disease was curable by either cod liver oil or by sunlight, but not by improved hygiene in the absence of these. The final unravelling of the mystery was to continue through the next few years, and a massive public health campaign in applying the findings lay ahead. In contrast to the previous failures, the story of the vanquishing of the disease is one of the most inspiring in the whole of nutritional history. By the 1940s, cases of rickets were a rarity—surely an outstanding achievement, and a fittingly triumphant note on which to finish a generally depressing chapter in the social history of Scotland.

8

FROM THE 1930s TO THE PRESENT

Better nutrition or worse?

The Scots nutrition expert Sir John Orr (later Lord Boyd Orr) wrote:

> The rapid advance in the science of nutrition in recent years has shown that the influence of diet on health and physique is profound. It has been proved that much of the ill-health which affects human populations can be attributed directly to deficiencies in diet.[1]

On the face of it, not a particularly earth-shattering statement— certainly not to us today, accustomed as we are to the idea that 'we are what we eat': in the 1930s, however, certainly quite a novel idea to the vast majority of people, for whom food might have represented variously a pleasant social custom, something to keep hunger at bay, or something in between these two extremes.

In the history of nutrition, the 1930s are a watershed, not least because of the publication of the Report (*Food, Health and Income,* 1936) from which the above statement is taken. This document must effectively have put paid to any undue complacency as to how well the nation was being fed at the time, for of all Boyd Orr's conclusions the most disturbing was that some 4.5 million people, representing 10 per cent of the UK population, were seriously under-nourished. Their diet, comprising principally cheap energy sources—bread, margarine, sugar, potatoes—was judged to be 'deficient in every constituent examined'. And in the children of this group he found widespread evidence of what he considered the three characteristic signs of malnutrition—rickets, bad teeth and anaemia.

Lord Boyd Orr, using data previously collected during a dietary survey of more than 1100 families in the UK, divided the population into six groups according to family income and food expenditure, and assessed the quality of the average diet in each. An estimate was made, too, of the supplies of the main foodstuffs in the country as a whole.

A close relationship emerged between family income and intakes of the 'protective foods'—milk, eggs, vegetables, fruit, butter, meats—although interestingly consumption of bread and potatoes remained remarkably constant in all. But only the top two income groups, representing some 30 per cent of the total population, were judged to have a surplus of those foods necessary for full health and wellbeing. (These figures refer of course to the UK as a whole: for Scotland, with her huge industrial area in the West in the grip of depression at the time, the picture was if anything even more gloomy.)

A daunting task, even in the light of today's knowledge, also undertaken by Lord Boyd Orr was an overall view of the nation's health. He found that there existed in Britain 'a great deal of preventable ill-health'; and he reached the firm conclusion that, as income increases, the incidence of disease declines, children grow more quickly, adult stature is greater, and general health and physique improve.

Today, dietary surveys on this scale are not unusual: in the 1930s they were still a novelty. Yet as early as 1881, a Committee of the British Association had actually published details of food consumption in Britain. Comparisons made by Boyd Orr with the 1930s showed that consumption of bread and potatoes had fallen by 30 per cent, that of meat had risen by 45 per cent, while the figures for butter and tea had doubled. By far the greatest dietary change, however, concerned sugar: in the hundred years up to 1936 consumption had multiplied no less than five times. And one other statistic startling to today's inflation-attuned reader is that from 1835 to 1936 the prices of bread and flour had remained virtually the same.

In the most recent chapters of this study we have concentrated almost exclusively upon the food of Scotland's poor industrial population, whereas we last looked at the diet of her agricultural workers—that plain but wholesome fare which had given rise to such a notably vigorous race—around the late eighteenth century, when those far-reaching developments leading eventually to industrial revolution were still in their infancy. The reason for this omission is simple. Rural diet had, surprisingly, remained substantially unchanged for that very lengthy period, some one-and-a-half centuries. True, by the nineteenth and early twentieth centuries meat had come to play, at least in some areas, a more important part. The old days of salt beef as an isolated winter feast were long past; many crofters now kept one or more pigs as well as their hens, while the more ready availability of firearms meant that game (hares, rabbits, venison) figured more frequently on the rural menu. In addition, braxy mutton (the flesh of sheep which had happened to die) was the shepherds' perquisite and formed a substantial part of their families' food. For the rest, however, the age-old diet prevailed, based predominantly on oats, barley, potatoes, dairy produce and eggs, with variable amounts of fish according to area; a diet with a very great deal to commend it nutritionally, apart from that traditional shortcoming—a generally poor representation of fruit and vegetables.

Just when this commendable state of affairs began to change is, as always with dietary changes, difficult to pinpoint. Change, however, it did, and in an important respect. As the horse-drawn carts (later replaced by vans) began to wend their way around the countryside, offering wares vastly more enticing than the home-grown products which had sufficed a simple and undemanding people, so the bad dietary habits of the industrial areas spread, and consumption of sugar and a variety of sweet foods, as well as of white flour and its products, rose steeply. On the credit side, however, fruit and vegetables were also becoming more widely available.

One pointer to the probable chronology of these events is the fact that in some Highland areas men formerly engaged in the milling of oats were no longer able to continue in that employment on their return from the First World War, so greatly decreased by then was the demand for oatmeal. In more isolated areas, on the other hand, the old staples—meal, potatoes, milk, fish—would continue to hold sway right up to the next war, twenty years later.

An elderly lady from the Outer Hebrides who kindly cast her mind back for the benefit of this study to the food of her childhood early this century, recalled that main meals in those days frequently centred around fish of one kind or another—salted herring or mackerel, dried salt fish, shellfish—although mutton, fowls and rabbits were also regular fare. Potatoes still formed a basic part of the food—not infrequently twice in the day—other vegetables apart from turnips being comparatively rare except in broth. Oats, Indian (maize) meal and flour, along with dairy produce, formed the basis of the other meals; puddings were almost exclusively rice and carrageen (purple seaweed); fruit remained almost as scarce as it had ever been. She recollected:

> The 'piece' we carried to school consisted of oatcakes or sometimes scones, with crowdie, treacle or jam. And well I remember how ravenous we always were by the time we had walked the long miles

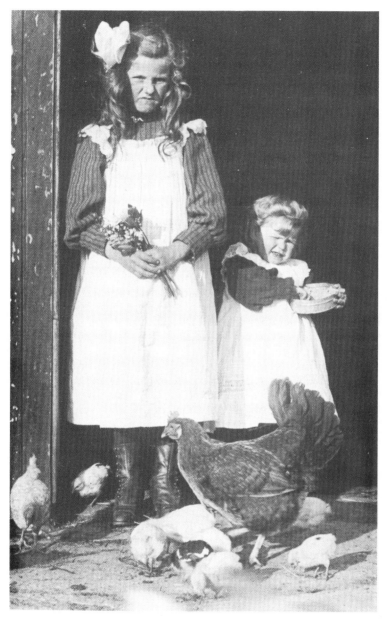

15   'Feeding the Hens', c. 1910. Photograph D Horne

home! A bottle of seal oil always stood on the mantelpiece and we seemed to be given a dose for every kind of ailment.

(If not the panacea the people believed it to be, this was doubtless an added protection against rickets—not that any such sign of deficiency was likely with a diet as sound as this.)

Despite a certain decline in some areas in the excellence of the rural diet by the 1920s, the findings of the Medical Research Council's Report No 101 (see Chapter 7) on the health of Scottish children in some of the agricultural counties was generally very favourable:

> The town children appeared to be poorly developed, often pale, and in Glasgow frequently rachitic, thus forming a striking contrast to the country children, who were sturdy, well-developed and rosy-cheeked, and in whom rickets was almost non-existent.

Their food, the researchers found, consisted of soups, stews, porridge, milk, oatcakes and scones, the cottage gardens contributing a limited variety of vegetables and some soft fruits. They noted the fact that although the parents were in general very poorly paid, they did at least have rent-free houses and received extras such as meal, potatoes and milk; fresh air and exercise were also duly acknowledged as having contributed to the altogether superior physique of the country children.

Personal recollections of schooldays in rural Inverness-shire during the 1930s and 1940s make the pursuit of the theme of the countryman's food of that period an easy task. By far the most interesting comparison which emerges, it now seems, is that between the lifestyle of the villagers living by the main road and that of the crofters living in relatively isolated situations (albeit in some cases less than a mile in actual distance) on the heights above the glen. Occasional childhood visits to these latter remain nostalgically clear in the memory. Even for children, there was a keen awareness of stepping back into an altogether older way of life. Was this because of the greater use of the Gaelic tongue, or the stoneflagged kitchen, or the kettle hanging by the swey over the open peat fire? More likely, perhaps, because of the tea-table, with its platter of large, thin, curling oatcakes, its girdle scones of surpassing lightness, spread with crowdie, heather honey or wild raspberry jam—all as welcome as the drink of milk warm from the cow emphatically was not. Down in the glen itself the inhabitants, amply served by the shops and vans, had long since succumbed to the lure of rolls, 'softies', and tea-breads, as well as to shop bread which was for the most part white, sometimes brown, and (if memory serves aright) almost never wholemeal. There too, all the same, a very strong baking tradition flourished—seldom, surely, can prizes offered by the popular Scottish Women's Rural Institute have been more hotly contested—although again the flour used was always white.

Cereal fibre content of the diet must have been relatively low. Nutritional standards in other respects were certainly high. Pre-war main meals were based predominantly on the cheaper cuts of meat, as well as hares, rabbits, fowls, mealy puddings. Fish appeared on the menu regularly (not, as might be supposed, as the result of poaching, but usually less colourfully by the van from Inverness). Eggs and cheese were prominent, as were fine home-made soups, milk and steamed puddings, stewed fruits and, in summer and autumn, an abundance of home-grown soft and hard fruits. Vegetable-growing was widespread, and the produce of high quality. Even if the range was fairly limited, at least the children were spared the challenge of eating spinach. Potatoes were as important as ever, most families having a 'drill' in a field as well as their quota from the garden, and no main meal was ever regarded as a 'right dinner' without this vital ingredient. Convenience foods were virtually unknown, the only exceptions, table jelly and tinned fruit or an occasional tin of tomato soup for Sunday dinner, being regarded as special treats.

It is doubtless significant that of all the inconveniences caused by the war—shortages of meat, bacon, cheese; the ubiquitous dislike of dried egg, and perpetual grumbles about the 'national' loaf—it was the rationing of sugar and sweet things which was felt by far the most keenly in the glen. Not, it should be added in fairness, that this reflects merely the communal sweet tooth: the sugar shortage inevitably hit hard in an area in which jam-making formed an important part of the traditional work-cycle. The larder with its neat rows of jars was a source of satisfaction and justifiable pride, jams being made largely from home-grown fruits—currants, gooseberries, rhubarb, apples, plums—or of wild fruits such as brambles and raspberries. The early weeks of the year, too, saw the bacon-cutter lent by a kindly shopkeeper going the rounds of the keen housewives as an aid to marmalade-making. To be deprived of all this was no small frustration to the glen folk. Despite assiduous fruit-bottling, and even repeated (abortive) attempts to produce an acceptable jam using saccharin and gelatine, effective use of the plentiful fruit crops remained a problem.

Up to the war various preserves—jams, jellies, honey,

marmalade, treacle, syrup—probably represented for most Highland people the principal source of sugar in the diet. Next came sugar taken in tea and cocoa (coffee being generally little used), while sweets, although undeniably popular, were for most restricted to a very few each week—usually for sustenance during the church sermon—while the consumption by children of a whole bar of chocolate at one time was certainly frowned on. In view of the disturbingly high incidence of overweight and even obesity among Scottish schoolchildren today it makes an interesting exercise to attempt an assessment of the probable sugar intake of a child in the above rural area just before the war compared with that of one at the present time.

Schoolchild, 1939

Sugar in various preserves	60g
tea and cocoa	30g
baked items and puddings	10g
sweets (occasional)	5g
	105g

Schoolchild, 1982

Sugar in cakes, plain and chocolate biscuits, puddings,	
tinned fruits	70g
sweets, chocolate, icecream, ice-lollies etc	70g
soft drinks	30g
preserves	30g
tea and coffee	25g
	225g

These examples have been calculated after careful consideration, and are believed to represent a true picture without exaggeration. The first is from personal childhood recollection and the second from repeated observation of the eating habits of Highland children today.

To return, however, from a necessarily lengthy digression along the path of rural dietary change, to the world of nutrition research in the years preceding the Second World War. So much was going on in the laboratory during the 1930s that in a general study of this type it becomes impossible to do more than touch upon it: research into the fascinating vitamins was of course proceeding apace, as was that of the role of the various inorganic elements in the diet of animals and humans.

In applied nutrition, we looked earlier at the researches of Lord Boyd Orr, and noted his concern at the generally low standard of nutrition among the poorer people in the whole of the country. At roughly the same time but many thousands of miles away, another outstanding nutritionist, this time an Irishman, was making his own unique contribution to nutritional knowledge. Sir Robert McCarrison, Director of Nutritional Research in India from 1927 to 1935,[2] was demonstrating, through prolonged animal feeding experiments, the close relationship between man and his food. His studies proved conclusively that good growth and physique are to be expected whenever food is fresh, whole (unprocessed) and grown on fertile soil, provided of course that a reasonably balanced diet is eaten. By feeding successive generations of rats on diets simulating those of different regions of India, he showed that both their physique and the incidence of disease corresponded with amazing accuracy to those of the peoples of those regions. In particular, he demonstrated the dire effects of a diet composed predominantly of refined carbohydrate, such as that of the rice-eating Bengalis—one which, clearly, had its counterpart in industrial Britain, and without any doubt in Scotland. It may be added that it is a measure of his standing as a pioneer in nutritional science that a society dedicated to his teaching—seeing nutrition as part of a far wider ecology—was formed in 1966 and flourishes today.

Experiments similar to McCarrison's were carried out in Scotland, and these too showed a striking divergence both in growth rates and mortality between rats fed on a poor diet and others whose food was supplemented with milk and green foods. More relevantly, a trial involving some 1500 Scottish primary schoolchildren, who were given extra milk at school over a period of seven months, demonstrated noticeable improvements in general health and vigour, and a mean increase in growth rate of around 20 per cent—findings which have been paralleled in many other places since that time.

A new era, however, was soon to begin. Few in the 1930s can surely have imagined how radically the whole scene was about to change; how quickly, for example, Boyd Orr's 'malnourished tenth' was to disappear, nor by what unwelcome means. But disappear it did soon after the start of what could be said to represent Britain's greatest-ever experiment in applied nutrition, the feeding of the nation during the 1939–45 war. That the experiment proved outstandingly successful was due to many factors, ranging from adequate scientific knowledge which enabled the Government (through the Medical Research Council) to formulate an efficient feeding policy, to the availability of a different, and perhaps typically British, talent—the administrative ability to ensure that the policy actually worked. Within a remarkably short time and with a few predictable exceptions, rich and poor found themselves eating substantially the same kind of food—a dietary uniformity, indeed, quite unique in the history of this country.

Well aware of the vital role of good nutrition in maintaining the full health and working efficiency of the population at a time when food supplies were likely to be severely curtailed, the Government introduced at an early stage certain key measures, in particular establishing a Ministry of Food whose task it was to ensure equitable distribution of supplies according to nutritional needs. Food subsidies were also introduced on a large scale to keep prices low. One important measure concerned the great British staple, bread. In Chapter 4, we saw how the 'pure food' protagonists had been campaigning for nearly a century for a higher-extraction (i.e. browner) loaf. Only now, because precious shipping space could no longer be used to bring from North America wheat of which a mere 70 per cent would be used for human food, was their dream realised. The extraction rate of flour was raised, so that the British people had a browner loaf whether they liked it or not; nor was white bread to re-appear until 1953.

The new 'national loaf' was fortified by the addition of calcium in the form of chalk, that mineral being less well absorbed from bread of higher extraction flour. The other great staple, margarine, was fortified by the addition of statutory amounts of the vitamins A and D, thus making it a more dependable year-round source of vitamin D than butter. These improvements in the nutritional value of bread and margarine represented a public health measure whose significance can scarcely be over-estimated.

An exhaustive account of all the measures affecting the Scottish diet during the war would be impossible in a general study of this kind. A brief look instead at the food fortunes of a typical Scots working family might not only prove more relevant but also demonstrate the very real beginnings of nutrition education for which wartime food policy was undoubtedly responsible.

The Macgregor family lived from 1939 to 1945 in Glasgow, where Mr Macgregor worked in an armaments factory. Although during this time food understandably played a fairly central part in their lives, they were by no means aware of all the measures being taken behind the scenes to ensure its supply; for example, while they immediately noticed the darker colour of the loaf (and did not like it) they were unaware of its added nutrients; nor did the familiar margarine, now vitaminised, seem in any way different. They used to the full all the foods which came under the 'straight' rationing scheme—fats, meat, bacon, sugar, cheese—including their small butter ration, although margarine had always previously sufficed; while their 'points' rations, covering such foods as preserves, sweets and dried fruits were carefully hoarded for special treats. Mrs Macgregor never missed any chance to join a queue for occasional luxuries such as oranges: like many another Scots housewife of the time, to whom poverty had previously been no stranger, she was enjoying the unaccustomed extra cash which full employment was making available. She was meticulous in securing the Welfare Foods—extra milk, concentrated orange juice and cod liver oil—to which her pre-school child was entitled as a member of a 'vulnerable group'. Gradually, too, she was becoming aware that some foods were considered more important than others for health. In the local Food Office prominent posters exhorted her to 'Go for Greens' and to give her family plenty of potatoes, so when, as part of the Dig for Victory campaign, her husband acquired an allotment and began to take pride in producing fine cabbages, cauliflowers, leeks and carrots, not a single one was ever wasted. Carrots were especially prized, since it was commonly reported that these—allegedly much used by night-fighter pilots—helped one to see in the dark. And when, due to the massive wartime increase in the number of industrial canteens, her husband was able to have a good midday meal at work, and the older children, following a similar expansion in the School Meals Service, began to enjoy having theirs in school, her task of feeding the family became very considerably lighter.

That thousands of industrial families like this one reached the end of the war a great deal better nourished than they had been before it, is attested by such indices as infant and maternal mortality rates and growth and dental health of children. Writing shortly after the war, Scots nutrition expert Dr Passmore was, surprisingly, able to state:

> There is ample evidence that the steady improvement in the health of young mothers, infants and children which began well before the war, has been maintained throughout the enormous difficulties and disturbances of war. Probably never before in history, and certainly not within living memory, have the children of Scotland been so healthy.[3]

This was surely a notable achievement. To the experts of the day the future must indeed have looked rosy enough—a beginning at least had been made on nutrition education: people now knew which foods were really important and which they could easily do without. Or did they? Time was to show, alas, that coping with food shortages was one thing; making a prudent choice from a wide variety of foods was quite another.

It might have seemed at least possible, for example, that most people after several years of fairly stringent rationing would have lost their proverbial sweet tooth. Not so, however. When the Ministry of Food removed sweets and chocolate from the ration, demand was immediately so overwhelming that they had to go sharply into reverse. Perhaps the main (if still minor) obvious change was that many people—arguably, for the most part the female of the species—had stopped taking sugar in their tea. As for fats, it is perhaps scarcely surprising that a nation so long deprived of these—and of the culinary delights which depend upon them—should by now be clamouring for more fatty and oily foods. A few years after the war, comparative studies carried out on the pre-war and post-war diets of UK working families showed that actual food habits had changed disappointingly little. Although there was some improvement in the nutritional value of their food, this was found to be due to the welfare foods and to the hidden fortification of bread and margarine rather than to any real change in food choice.

All of this was merely a foretaste of what was to follow. Rationing did not end completely until 1954. By the end of that decade, Scotland was launched on an eating and drinking spree which, at least for a great many, still continues unabated. This kind of pattern is by no means unique to Scotland. It is recognised that, with growing affluence, intakes of meats, fats and sweet foods increase, while consumption of the cheaper bread and potatoes falls. Generally, however, the increased energy intakes following such changes are not offset by increased energy expenditure. And this has, of course, one unfortunate, predictable consequence, to which Scotland has surely proved no exception—that people become fat.

From the end of the war onwards, any attempt to present a tidy, chronological picture of anything which could be termed 'the Scots diet' becomes virtually impossible. In every direction, the whole field of food and health was expanding. On the research side, a great variety of subjects were being studied. While some researchers were turning their attention to the nutritional requirements of laboratory animals and farm livestock, others were busily determining the needs of human infants, toddlers, schoolchildren, adolescents, pregnant women, old people. Energy expenditure was studied for a wide range of activities, from the ordinary and homely (like ironing, or scrubbing a floor) to the more rarified (like playing a Beethoven sonata on the piano). Meanwhile, at the eating end of the spectrum, food habits changed at an unprecedented rate. Growing affluence and greatly increased opportunities for travel were widening the horizons of many Scots. Freezer ownership, too, had begun to increase; and as more and more housewives went to work outside the home, there developed an ever-increasing demand for the bewildering array of convenience foods which an expanding food technology industry was able to bring to the shelves of the supermarkets. With a scene so complex, therefore, it is feasible here to take but a brief look at the main topics of dietary interest, and attempt to pinpoint the main trends which have characterised this period.

Somewhere around 1960, the dietary scene began to be dominated by a single concern which had never given trouble on any large scale before. A nutrition expert had just coined a new phrase which would be heard a great deal—'the malnutrition of affluence'. It is possibly difficult even for today's younger health professionals to appreciate fully just what a new idea this was to the majority at that time. Malnutrition from *under*-nourishment, yes: this conjured up a picture of emaciated, pot-bellied children in the deprived areas of the world. But that malnutrition could arise in times of plenty from a wrong choice of food, and especially from too much food, and that it could bring in its wake a disturbing number of very real health problems, was indeed a new thought for most Scots people. They had to begin to learn that carrying an extra load of weight could put a serious strain on their bodies—and not just on joints, but on heart and blood-vessels as well.

As the food manufacturers were moving in to provide the Scots with a wide-ranging variety of the sugary, starchy, fatty foods they craved, so the experts on diet—geared previously to teaching people how to obtain *enough* of the various nutrients—began their campaign to remove the offending extra pounds. And while some of those afflicted contented themselves with dropping an artificial sweetener into their coffee at the end of an ample meal, the more determined dieters set themselves to endure the rigours of an ever-increasing number of reducing regimes—if not the conventional calorie-restricted diets of the hospital-based clinics, then, as likely as not, the Bananas and Milk Diet, the Two by Two Diet, the Mini-C Diet, the Swedish Milk Diet, even, at one time, the Yes You Can Diet. The media joined enthusiastically in the campaign, with television (itself contributing to the problem by decreasing the energy output of those who sat, often for hours, watching it), plugging various slimming products among the advertisements for mouth-watering, high energy foods; while no woman's magazine was seemingly complete without its quota of recipes, slimming hints, or photographs of various slimmers before and after their personal (successful) battle.

Sugar consumption, no doubt due to all of the above, has been falling since 1960: it should be added, however, that this is true only of sugar as such, and not of the many products in which it is concealed. Unfortunately bread also came to be associated wrongly with sugar as a 'bad' food, producing only 'empty calories'.

As more and more avenues began to be explored, treatments ranged from vibrator belts, sauna baths and jogging at one end of the spectrum to appetite-reducing drugs and bulking agents in foods at the other; or even, in the intractable cases, to hospital treatment involving periods of fasting, surgical removal of fat, or wiring of the jaw to decrease food intakes. Group therapy in the form of slimming clubs began to be practised in many places, and by the end of the 1960s the commercial slimming organisations were set fair to become very big business indeed. While cookery books had never been glossier or more popular, so too books on the ever-topical subject of slimming proliferated as never before. Glasgow physiologist/nutritionist Professor John Durnin summed up the situation amusingly:

> The weight of written material on slimming, if distributed and carried around by all the obese people in the world, would increase their energy expenditure enough to slim them in a couple of weeks.[4]

Even babies, it seemed, were by no means immune to the harmful effects of current dietary excesses. By the beginning of the 1970s it was becoming apparent that the plump, bonny babies who won the prizes at the local baby show were not necessarily the healthiest, and that there were far too many plump babies. Not only were fat deposits being laid down which it was feared might last for life; doctors were also becoming alarmed by some of the other serious effects of over-concentrated feeding. A vigorous health education campaign was therefore launched to alert mothers to the potential dangers and instruct them in correct feeding techniques, particular emphasis being laid upon avoidance of an early taste for sweet things, as well as on breast-feeding—a practice which had been declining for several decades—as the ideal. That this latter aspect at least was having a successful outcome is attested by a distinct upward trend in the popularity of breast-feeding ever since that time.

But a new and altogether more serious aspect of over-nutrition had, by around the mid 1950s, begun to cause deep concern. The incidence of coronary heart disease—that type of heart condition which is due to a decreased supply of blood to the heart, and which can cause a heart attack—was rising steadily, and would eventually reach epidemic proportions. In those early days, few could have guessed at the massive search which lay ahead to ascertain its cause, nor how highly controversial its nature would be.

At the time, research was centred upon the hypothesis—for which wholly convincing evidence never was to be forthcoming—that dietary fat, and particularly saturated (hard) fat of animal origin, was the culprit. Later, following the realisation that coronary heart disease results from an interplay of several factors, the net was flung wider—to take in, for example, sugar and other refined carbohydrates, excessive smoking, inactivity, stress, soft water and various genetic factors.

Throughout the 1950s and 1960s research spread worldwide as medical researchers tirelessly investigated the food habits, lifestyle and health status of milk-drinking African camel-drivers or fat-chewing Eskimos or fish-eating Japanese fishermen; or, nearer home, studied the influence of exercise, stress and food on London bus-drivers and conductors; or compared the health fortunes of a large number of pairs of Irish brothers whose ways had diverged, one having remained in agricultural Ireland while the other had emigrated to an industrial life in the USA.

Out of the ensuing welter of statistics no clear pattern emerged. Medical scientists, at no time renowned for unanimity of opinion, were sharply divided in their interpretation of the results. Many advised strict reduction of those foods containing cholesterol—a fatty substance found in the deposits clogging the arteries of those affected—and of animal fats; at the same time advocating increased intakes of the polyunsaturated fats—oils produced from various plants and seeds—which advice, predictably, caused an unprecedented boom in sales of vegetable oils and a threat to the production of such foods as cholesterol-rich eggs. Other equally reputable experts, on the other hand, deplored the loss of the valuable dairy and meat products, and even the seemingly univers-ally-growing distaste for fat meat. And yet others were convinced that most of the blame should not be attributed to fat at all, but to sugar and its multiple products, along with the refined, highly pro-cessed foods which have come to be accepted in modern industrial societies.

While, through the seventies, the sometimes bitter controversy went on, huge numbers of people in Britain, principally men in the 45–65 age-group, continued to die of coronary disease. Once again, Scotland was finding herself high in an altogether unenviable league table, vying with Finland and Northern Ireland for top place. The British Regional Heart Study, investigating such diverse factors as drinking water, climate, air pollution and blood groups, identified the West of Scotland as the region with the highest mortality from the disease—from which, to quote a random example, 156,000 in England and Wales, and proportionately more in Scotland, died in 1976.

In the absence of clear proof of their efficacy, most dietary regimes restricting cholesterol were being abandoned by the 1980s, a change which must have caused mixed feelings in those who for years had had to avert their eyes from their favourite butter, or make do with milk on their strawberries. While research evidence continued to be conflicting and medical opinion remained divided, it began to look as if the lowering of blood levels of cholesterol—which is formed within the body as well as being provided by certain foods—did not necessarily afford protection against the disease. Most surprising of all, some reputable authorities suggested that the dread cholesterol might even be a protective mechanism against other diseases.

One thing at least seemed to be indisputable. Coronary heart disease, like obesity, is not found among those whose lifestyle is frugal, but is a scourge of affluent industrialised societies. Essentially it has to do with too-muchness. One journalist put it like this: 'Our so-called higher living standards, leading to over-indulgence in food, tobacco and alcohol, coupled with a reluctance to walk instead of ride, are leading many of us to an early grave.'[5] Accordingly, most advice began to centre upon the avoidance of overweight, using energy-restricted diets; along with control of blood pressure levels, avoidance of smoking, and emphasis on taking a prudent amount of exercise.

All of the foregoing might well give rise to the impression that the entire post-war era has been characterised exclusively, nutritionally speaking, by a campaign to combat the ill effects of over-indulgence. On the contrary, however, during these years there has been much concern over the needs of a considerable number of people whose condition remains an exception to the generally high living standards—for example the rising numbers of unemployed people, as well as the aged, the one-parent families, the disabled, the larger and poorer families and the socially inadequate.

Many health professionals campaigned vigorously against the cuts in welfare foods brought into force in the early 1970s, fearing that health improvements of past decades might be allowed to lapse. More than one dietary survey, indeed, has demonstrated that there are considerable numbers of children at risk of undernutrition from one cause or another: such children often experience educational difficulties through being generally less alert than those of higher nutritional status.

In the same period it also became a matter of some urgency to identify the dietary needs of a growing geriatric population. In Scotland, the award of Glasgow's St Mungo prize to the renowned pioneer geriatrician Sir Ferguson Anderson was a pointer to the importance then attached by the authorities to this vital branch of health care. In stating that elderly people are prone to suffer from various degrees of undernutrition or malnutrition—due perhaps to apathy through loneliness, or health problems, unsuitable housing or immobility—one is obviously aware that in fact there exists no homogeneous group to be known conveniently as the elderly. Instead, there are alert and sprightly eighty year-olds who are able to cope remarkably well, and apathetic seventy year-olds who are not. Although meals on wheels, lunch clubs, over-sixties groups, home helps, day-care centres and sheltered housing have all become an accepted part of community care in recent decades, occasional tragic cases of neglect have continued to stab the public conscience; nor can it truly be said that in this area either undernutrition or frank deficiency states are yet things of the past.

One condition which still occurs widely among older folk is simple iron-deficiency anaemia. Another is bone disease of nutritional origin: osteomalacia (the adult form of rickets) was recently stated to be still a widespread condition. Not surprisingly in view of the important part played by sunshine in prevention of rickets, it has been discovered that the disease occurs primarily in those who are shut-ins because of immobility—often through being unsuitably housed—rather than in those elderly folk who have rather aptly been described as free-range.

Nor have the elderly been the only group affected. In view of the outstandingly successful campaign waged in earlier decades against the old, old enemy of Scotland's children, the re-appearance of rickets in Glasgow around 1960 (although admittedly not in its previous severe form) was especially disturbing. While in these cases infantile rickets tended to be found in white children, the much larger number of older children and even adolescents affected belonged to the immigrant Asian population. During the years

1968–78, during which Glasgow's Asian population increased from 8,000 to 14,000, no fewer than 138 Asians were discharged from hospital with a diagnosis of either nutritional rickets or osteomalacia: in the same period, the incidence of rickets in the white population was extremely low. A vigorous health education campaign subsequently launched (with the aid of Asian community leaders) employed every kind of technique, including a specially-made film, in an all-out effort to increase intakes of the vital vitamin D: supplements of the vitamin were offered free of charge upon demand for the children of all ethnic groups under five, and all Asians under 18. Nevertheless, the amount of vitamin D in food was clearly not the whole story. The fact that intakes in those affected were not always lower than those of healthy people pointed to exposure to sunlight as a critical factor. Another aspect was the preponderance of wholemeal chappati flour in the Asian diet, with the possibility that, given an already borderline vitamin D intake, its absorption was being adversely affected by the high-fibre flour.

That this last point should not be unduly emphasised, however, but rather that any neccessary correction should be made by achieving safe intakes of vitamin D, was becoming clear as, from around 1970, another pronounced dietary deprivation of twentieth century industrial man was being exposed. Researches carried out in different countries, notably by Mr D P Burkitt,[6] a surgeon, were demonstrating that lack of dietary fibre could be considered an important factor in a wide range of human disorders. His studies among some tribal communities in Africa, for example, had shown these people, whose food consisted principally of unrefined cereals and plant foods, to be remarkably free from diseases common in industrialised societies. Not only did this list include dental decay, obesity, gall-bladder disease and diabetes; it also extended to bowel conditions such as constipation, appendicitis, diverticular disease, haemorrhoids and, most serious of all, bowel cancer. (Of this last, Scotland has one of the highest rates in the world.) In a sense, a relative freedom from these among primitive peoples could be said to have been predictable; nor was it altogether surprising to find for instance that in black and white Americans the incidence of such disorders was relatively equal. What really was perplexing was the seeming immunity of these tribal people to diseases of the circulation—varicose veins, hypertension, deep vein thrombosis, coronary heart disease—this last of course of maximum interest in the light of the coincidental massive search for its cause. As with black and white Americans, it became clear that the incidence of the above diseases increases when lifestyle (and diet) become westernised.

A spate of research followed—the findings not necessarily in accord on every point—which led to a fairly widespread belief that dietary fibre should be considered a potent factor in the prevention of disease. All of this appeared to be merely confirming what other medical researchers had been at pains to point out many years before. For example, back in the 1920s and 1930s Sir Robert McCarrison had been highlighting those diseases which he believed to be due to modern man's dependence on over-refined foods. And from the 1930s onward Surgeon Captain T L Cleave had been condemning what he saw clearly as the ravages of excessive consumption of sugar, white bread and other fibre-depleted foods.

More attention was being paid to constipation—sometimes referred to as the 'secret national problem'—which some estimated to be affecting around 50 per cent of the entire population (and to be costing something in the order of £10m annually in laxatives). For a very long time the cereal fibre content of the British diet had been falling; first, through the gradual reduction in the extraction rate of flour for bread-making, from an original wholemeal 100 per cent (i.e. using every part of the wheat grain) to around 80–85 per cent (a brownish loaf) and finally to white flour at 70–72 per cent. In modern times not only had refined packaged cereals largely replaced porridge for breakfast, but consumption of bread itself was continuing to fall; while surveys showed that the vast majority still preferred white bread, a smaller number choosing a range of brown loaves and by far the smallest number the wholemeal variety. Although during the past 100 years consumption of fruit and vegetables had generally risen greatly, this had been less true in Scotland: in any case, the fibre from this source was found to be a less effective laxative than that from cereals (and to a lesser extent also than that of root vegetables and pulses).

While one expert talked of modern man's 'over-paid body and under-worked gut',[7] in 1977 a leading article in the *British Medical Journal*,[8] taking a somewhat amused look at the new dietary vogue, pointed out that the developed world, in discovering fibre (which is simply the cell walls of plants and the very basis of life on this planet), is at last waking up to its removal from food somewhere in its journey from field to shop.

As a consequence of all the publicity accorded to the new teaching, a number of Scots did begin to return to a greater use of their native cereal, oats. More marked, however, was the effect of the health-food movement in persuading more people to use wholemeal bread and other whole foods. A far greater number of Scots with bowel disorders, however, found it simpler to retain their life-long food habits but to sprinkle bran on to those very cereals from which it had been removed—a somewhat paradoxical situation. Indeed, it is arguable that some came to regard bran as a substance to be sprinkled on to food rather than as a component of food at all.

More recent teaching has set out to correct attitudes to all of this. The experts stress that adding fibre to an otherwise unchanged diet is merely one side of the coin: dietary starch must be eaten, not in an unnaturally refined state, but along with its *natural* complement of fibre. It is not a simple lack of fibre, but over-consumption of fibre-depleted foods, which leads to the 'diseases of civilisation'.

In this overall study only brief mention can be made of those other problems—some directly dietary, others of merely fringe concern—which have been engaging the attention of health professionals during the past couple of decades. For one thing, dental health was causing much concern—an estimate in the mid 1970s, for example, stating that nearly half of the entire population over the age of sixteen had no teeth of their own at all. Fluoridation of water supplies as a preventive measure in tooth decay was, and remains, a highly emotive issue. While much medical and dental opinion supports the measure, other reputable doctors and scientists hold grave doubts as to its wisdom. It may seem superfluous to point out that the health of teeth is more sensibly protected by a good diet than by any other means.

Deep concern has been expressed by a growing number of health experts over the potential ill effects of a very wide range of latter-day hazards including pesticides and weedkillers, antibiotics used in livestock rearing, radiation, and industrial pollutants such as lead and mercury. While these, clearly, are outwith the scope of this study, there are other concerns which do deserve mention. The pioneer work of Dr Richard Mackarness in the field of food allergies is now well known. In Scotland today, too, important research is being undertaken by Dr Ian Menzies in Dundee into the food and chemical sensitivities of disturbed children, something which surely deserves serious attention in view of the eating habits of many young people today. Another important area of research is the study of suspected links between poor maternal nutrition and serious congenital defects, such as spina bifida, incidence of which is disturbingly high in the so-called Celtic areas, including Scotland. Yet another field of study whose importance cannot be over-estimated is that which concerns environmental effects (obviously including the diet) on the development of cancer.

Undernutrition and malnutrition in various forms still exist in

Scotland today. There are for example many poor children whose intakes of the valuable foods are low, who are well below average in height, and whose health certainly gives no cause for complacency; thousands who habitually eat no breakfast, and whose food is predominantly of the junk variety. Many old folk are still at risk of malnutrition to a greater or lesser degree. Yet from the foregoing it must be clear that a much greater number of health problems stem from over-consumption of food, and indeed of alcohol as well. In varying degrees, these problems are of course shared by the rest of the developed world.

In the period at which we have been looking, more and more millions of men, women and children, especially children, in the rest of the world have suffered from every kind of nutritional deficiency, or have died of starvation.

9

THE PRESENT POSITION

What are the nutritional problems?

The deluge of dietary advice—much of it conflicting—which has been directed at the public over the past couple of decades from a wide variety of sources has led to such a distinct loss of credibility that one hesitates to offer a personal contribution. On the other hand, any review of the Scots diet which aims to be purely historical and objective, and offers neither personal observations, criticisms nor recommendations could justifiably be said to lack a cutting edge.

For a long time now the statement has been repeated over and over again that diet has a profound effect upon health. Many have been at pains to point out that man has no inbuilt sense of how to choose his food wisely, nor does increasing affluence necessarily mean improved nutrition—or better health. But does anybody really believe this? The implications of such assertions are surely far-reaching and profound. Yet nutrition teaching still comes far down the list of priorities in health education, not to mention the curriculum of our medical schools; while preventive medicine is still too often seen primarily as catching things in time through improved screening techniques, rather than as true prevention—which ought surely at least to include persuading the population to eat a health-producing diet. Nor can it easily be denied that both agriculture and the gigantic food industry are still run for profit rather than for health.

In this study, a fairly close look has been taken at the Scots diet with its traditional strengths and weaknesses. In the case of the weaknesses, we have noted the social deprivation which initially fostered them, in particular the clamour for cheap food sources which led in time to the insidious take-over by sugar and white flour, and eventually a host of products based on these.

One is often asked how good—or more often, how bad—the Scots diet is today. In attempting to answer this question it is as well to keep two points in mind—first, that there has been no such thing as 'the Scots diet' since urban and rural so disastrously parted company back around 1800 (see Chapter 6); secondly, the complexity of modern food habits makes it extremely difficult for even a full-time researcher, and probably presumptuous for anyone else, to risk making generalisations.

Obviously, while it is tempting to enlarge on the dismal side, one is really seeking to present the most balanced picture possible. From the positive angle, therefore, I believe a considerable number of Scottish families today to be very well fed indeed. Thousands of housewives are more nutrition-conscious than they ever were before. More and more are baking their own bread, and making use of wholemeal flour, as well as oatmeal, pulses and other whole foods, a trend which clearly owes much to the health/whole foods movement. Some are growing a considerable part of their own food, and becoming more adventurous, for example, in the range of vegetables they use. Many, on the other hand, remain true to traditional dishes like broths, porridge, mealy puddings and oat-cakes. (Tune in, for instance, to one of Radio Scotland's phone-in programmes on traditional cookery, and the range of knowledge and practice of the old skills will soon become apparent.) It should certainly be noted, too, that there are definite signs of the food industry in Scotland beginning to move forward in response to new, enlightened demands.

Finally, in pursuit of a balanced picture of food habits in Scotland today we would do well to remember that, while deep concern rightly prevails over the ravages of those 'diseases of civilisation' attendant upon affluence and over-nutrition, there are also other ills with which, thankfully, we no longer have to contend. Not only has the infant mortality rate fallen fairly steadily since the beginning of the century; there is evidence too that today's more ample diet affords protection against old scourges like tuberculosis, as well as the more serious effects of virus infections. If we look, for example, at measles—to us a fairly routine childhood infection on the whole—we find that among the poor in the developing world this is a killer disease.

During the past few years I can claim to have discussed diet with a considerable number of people. Apart from professional colleagues, these have been for the most part groups of housewives who have invited me to speak on this theme; and they have represented varied backgrounds, coming predominantly from urban Strathclyde or rural Tayside. Looking back, it is remarkable how many expressed concern about current dietary trends. Many mothers (and grandmothers) voiced their anxiety over the food preferences of their children; in particular, those whose offspring had weight problems pointed out how strongly various social pressures militate against dieting attempts—the school tuckshops, the ice-cream vans, the TV advertisements, the traditional Scots habit of giving children gifts of sweets. Some clearly felt that food habits had taken a wrong turning since the last war; others, that we have been taken over by an increasingly sophisticated food industry, so that more and more young folk are substituting highly processed foods for fresh, wholesome products.

It could be argued that such views are not truly representative, since the women concerned belonged mainly to Women's Rural Institutes or Women's Guilds and were for the most part middle-aged or older. Even so, they do at least indicate that it is not only the cranks who feel stirrings of unease at what has been happening to the diet in Scotland for some time.

Still, it may well be argued, is the same thing not happening all over the developed world? Are things here any worse than, say, in England? Unfortunately, not only is our health record worse, but market research has repeatedly indicated that our food habits are too. As recently as mid-1982, a survey of the (supermarket) buying habits of 6,000 housewives in the UK demonstrated that, compared to housewives South of the Border, the Scots use significantly more tinned meats and vegetables, especially peas and beans; more tinned soups, pastas and wrapped bread; more syrup and treacle; more buns, cakes, pies and biscuits.

Possibly the following real-life examples may serve more effectively than mere theoretical discussion to illustrate harmful food trends in Scotland.

At a recent confererence which I attended in one of Scotland's new towns, the venue was a young people's residential hostel. No cook was employed, allegedly because it was found cheaper to use convenience foods. The unvarying daily menu therefore was as follows:

Breakfast	(Refined) cereals, milk and sugar; sliced white bread, with individually-packed portions of butter and jelly marmalade.
Lunch and Dinner	Packet soup; ready-frozen meals— sliced roast meat, peas, mashed potatoes; ice-cream and tinned fruit cocktail.
Snacks	Coffee and sweet biscuits.

Perhaps even more surprising than the almost total absence of fresh and fibrous foods was the frequently voiced comment of several fellow-guests as to how good the food was.

This is of course no isolated instance, but simply one example of a trend which many in this country have come to accept unquestionably today. In the local supermarket of my home town, it requires no particularly diet-orientated eye to notice neighbouring trolleys devoid of fresh foods but laden with such items as sugar and syrup, lemonade and coke, packet and tinned soups, readycooked pasta snacks, cakes, chocolate biscuits, crisps and sweets.

A few years ago a Dane, Paul Stemann, wrote a most interesting account of his trek across the Highlands with a pack pony. While he greatly appreciated the people and the superb scenery, his comments on the food were less than complimentary. He missed nothing—the tired vegetables in the shops, the general lack of well-cultivated gardens on the West coast—but especially he wondered why it was that fresh food seemed to play such a small part in the daily menus. 'All through the Highlands', he writes, 'there were venison, salmon, lobster, crab, wild raspberries, rowanberries, chanterelles—all the most delectable foods. It was all around, but never put in front of you.'[1]

The sweet-eating habit of large numbers of Scottish children is so well known that it is probably superfluous to underline it. Here, however, is a true recent example. In a local sweet-shop a friend waited while a family of three children made their selection. When they had left, she remarked in surprise to the shop assistant that they had disposed of £1. 'Oh, that's nothing,' was the reply, 'these three usually have a fiver to spend on sweets.'

Lack of fresh foods must cause particular concern in the case of children. Various health professionals have reported interviewing schoolchildren whose habitual daily menu consisted roughly of the following: one or two packets of crisps for breakfast (or quite often no breakfast at all); pastries or rolls for lunch (a West of Scotland special is a roll or Vienna loaf filled with chips); sweets and coke on the way home from school; and for dinner, a sausage roll, bridie or pie with chips, followed perhaps by bought fruit pie or trifle, or jelly or ice-cream. Some years ago, it has to be admitted, I might have been content to calculate from food tables the nutritional value of any person's meals, and to accept them as satisfactory if the totals reached recommended levels. Today the number of artificial additives—colourings, preservatives, flavourings, sweeteners—would be more likely to engage my attention.

But quite apart from concern about either poor dietary quality or potentially high intakes of artificial additives, it must immediately be obvious that eating in this way is expensive. At a time when the rate of unemployment is so high—to mention only a single aspect—this is surely undesirable. It stands to reason that the more foods one buys which have been prepared and packaged, the more one is paying towards the cost of such processing rather than for the foods themselves.

In Chapter 8 we looked at the way in which the quality of the diet in rural Scotland, once so admirable, gradually declined to reach a level not substantially different from that of the industrial population. What about the industrial diet itself? How has it changed—for example since before the Second World War? An interesting comparison emerges from Molly Weir's vivid account of her Glasgow childhood in *Shoes Were for Sunday*:

> Poverty is a very exacting teacher, and I had been well taught. We learned never to waste a single thing during our childhood. We knew food wasn't always there for the asking, and we learned to know the price and value of everything. I discovered that a high-priced roast wasn't necessarily better than the delicious potted meats Grannie could make with the cheaper shin of beef. By the time I was 10 years old, Grannie could trust me to choose a piece of beef, knowing I'd bring back the very best value in the shop for the money I had to spend.[2]

While nobody is likely to suggest that the city diet of the time was in any way exemplary, one sentence certainly stands out: 'We learned never to waste a single thing.' To what extent has comparative affluence eroded the once proverbial Scottish virtue of thrift? Perhaps the dustmen can best answer that question. Certainly it is no easy task to carry out actual surveys of food waste, since the very awareness of being observed obviously influences family habits.

Molly Weir's account raises some other questions too: for example, are there still grannies like hers around today—skilled in basic household economy, able to teach such good sense to their grand-daughters? And the children of the tenements—are they still as budget-conscious as they were? How many of today's city housewives would be likely to produce the tasty potted meats (or jams and jellies, scones and pancakes, home-made vegetable soups) in which her grandmother took such pride? Probably the answer to all these questions is that there must be some who are still as skilled, but a great many more who are not.

It is all a measure of how greatly times have changed. Thankfully, relatively few have to watch every single penny quite so carefully as in the days of which Molly Weir writes. Another social change has been in the number of women who now work outside the home, and who would quite rightly retort that they have no time to make their own soups or bake their own scones. Certainly time can, today, be for many more valuable than money. And lastly, there exists nowadays a food industry whose business it is to apply that technology which no longer takes place in the kitchen. This particular social change is well illustrated by Molly Weir when she describes those rare occasions on which her aunt would send her out to buy sixpenceworth of cooked peas. 'H'm—paying good money to get someone else to do your cooking for you', her grandmother would snort. 'But that', continues the author, 'was exactly what our depraved tastes enjoyed.' For the record, it may be added that, to her obvious delight, the cooked-food ban did not extend to chips.

So could we manage without our food industry today? Pursuing a balanced view, we would surely have to answer no, not by any stretch of the imagination. In our predominantly urban society, a great deal of our food must be preserved and stored for varying periods of time. However much we might wish that everybody could have the pleasure of picking their own peas—or cauliflowers or leeks or raspberries—fresh on the day of eating, for a great many city-dwellers this is simply not possible. This is not to say that large numbers could not, for instance, be urged to buy far more fruit and vegetables in the fresh state, nor that many suburban and even country people could not grow much more of their own food than they do now. At the same time it might be as well to dispel the commonly-held notion that all food which is not fresh is necessarily in all respects inferior. Indeed, I clearly remember occasions years ago, on which random testing demonstrated in frozen green vegetables (which, for freezing, have to be of high quality) higher contents of vitamin C than those present in similar fresh products culled from shops with a slowish turnover. Vitamin C is, of course, highly destructible and its presence therefore as good a barometer of quality as any. Which, again, is not to say that for a growing number of people today, including the writer, choice would not emphatically fall on fresh, organically-grown produce on every possible occasion.

It will be realised, then, that concern stems much less from this kind of processing—at least, provided that the methods used are carefully selected with maximum nutritional safeguards in mind—than from the seemingly endless range of convenience foods, generally with high contents of sugar or salt, refined cereals, and a whole miscellany of artificial ingredients. Although some of these must doubtless be accepted as having a place in the housekeeping of the modern home (and few of us, surely, can claim *never* to use any of them) concern becomes very real in those cases in which, for one reason or another, there is dependence on a very narrow range of products, possibly even to the total exclusion of fresh food.

For some of us, too, the increasing use of what have been termed 'designed consumer foods' also raises questions. In these, the basic raw material—be it potato or cereal—has been so changed as to render it unrecognisable. Each year an astronomical sum is spent in the UK on potato crisps. It would be a brave person indeed (even in a dietetic household) who would dare cast aspersions on such highly popular fare: in any case, not only are crisps preferable to sweets, but surely some 'food for fun' must be allowed. Nothing is more boring to children than 'eat it because it's good for you'. But two wishes might perhaps be expressed. One, that crisps should not usurp the place of meals; the other, that some at least of these vast stocks of potatoes might be diverted to produce, instead, delicious hot baked potatoes—which were long ago sold on Scotland's city streets. The emergence of a growing number of small restaurants selling jacket potatoes is a welcome development: the more young people are introduced to real food, the better.

All of the foregoing has concentrated on the deficiencies in the diet of many Scots today, as well as on the superfluity of processed foods containing sugar and refined starch: in contrast, the tendency to choose meals high in fat is probably less often emphasised. Yet, especially in view of recent research linking certain forms of cancer with high fat intakes, this is a fault which certainly ought to be stressed.

Again, a real-life example may be useful. Recently in a well-known Tayside restaurant my husband and I were served a delicious meal of fresh salmon, generously garnished with anchovy butter and accompanied by several salads in a rich mayonnaise, followed by a fruit tart almost entirely filled with whipped cream. Out of interest I decided to calculate the estimated fat content of the meal, and found it to be something around double our *daily* requirement—no wonder we felt satiated for the rest of that day! While this could be said to be fairly typical of many up-market meals, calculation of the top favourite high tea of bacon, sausage, egg and chips reaches a fat total not far short of these. (Many people, too, are possibly unaware of the hidden fat which can be added by such items as cakes, shortbread, doughnuts and chocolate biscuits.)

Finally, it has to be said that many in Scotland today simply eat too much of everything—not that this is a problem by any means confined to this country alone. Nor is it confined to any one social group. This first became clear to me, I believe, during an unusually prolonged industrial strike in the mid-1970s when the wives of some strikers (in the Strathclyde area) shared details of their normal food budgets in a local newspaper. Not only were the amounts of butcher meat, bacon and sausages, eggs, butter, and baked and canned goods of staggering proportions: it emerged quite clearly that these ample providers were mothers who sincerely believed in 'feeding the family well'. Since that time, many thousands of Scots have joined the dole queue, and would no longer be able to eat in this way even if they wanted to. But it can be said with certainty that there are still far too many who do habitually over-eat, and that of these a considerable number may well do so because they honestly believe this to be the right way for health. And for this misconception, those of us who claim to be nutrition experts must surely bear much of the blame.

Nutrition is still a comparatively new branch of knowledge and one of which we are learning more all the time. That some mistakes have been made cannot be denied. And while teaching has had to change course at times, it would surely have been worse never to admit to being wrong at all! Taken all in all, it has to be said that much confusion currently exists as to what is the best way of eating for health. A leading nutrition authority, Dorothy Hollingsworth,[3] writing on this very subject, takes bread as an example. 'Why do many people think bread contains nothing but starch, and that starch is more fattening than fat, sugar or alcohol?' she asks. 'Our communication and education about nutrition and diet must have been at fault if so many people have got this faulty idea.' Yes, it has indeed been at fault, largely perhaps because after the years of wartime stringency, dietitians were at pains to teach the public how to obtain *enough* nutrients—enough protein, enough minerals, enough vitamins—although interestingly, possibly the only factor which was not stressed sufficiently is today's must, dietary fibre! Miss Hollingsworth continues:

> Such advice was good when money or food or both were short, but . . . it was not thought necessary to teach moderation, or that the balance of energy input and output is probably of paramount importance. The would-be educators did not really have the chance to observe that the majority of people, if given freedom of choice as in a present-day supermarket, and sufficient money, do not have adequate knowledge to spend their money with total nutritional wisdom.

So we find ourselves faced with the major problem of overweight and its consequences for health—some of them, especially in later life, serious. How widespread is this problem in Scotland today? Accurate overall figures would be difficult to produce, but it has lately been suggested, for instance, that as many as 65 per cent of adult females and 35 per cent of males are overweight. Obviously it would be unfair to give the impression that all overweight persons are gluttonous or, at least in certain cases, noticeably greedier than their slimmer, more fortunate neighbours!

Looking in the previous chapter at current health problems, we noted not only the high incidence of coronary heart disease but also a whole range of digestive disorders including peptic ulcer, constipation, diverticulitis and gall-bladder disease, as well as the alarmingly high incidence of bowel cancer. On the reverse side we mentioned some of the ills to which the under-nourished in our society may be prone. That all of this adds up to an impressive amount of ill-health few would deny. What by no means all health professionals are agreed upon, not surprisingly, is the extent to which faulty dietary habits can be blamed for it. With some disorders, implication of dietary factors is clear; with others, although conclusive evidence is not yet available, circumstantial evidence is nevertheless strong. It would be true to say, however, that the number of those who are persuaded of the vital importance of good diet is growing steadily.

Changing eating habits is by no means easy, as all will testify who have made the attempt. Generally people tend to resist any idea that their food habits are at fault, preferring on the whole to believe that a little of what you fancy does you good. Still, it is obvious that somehow a beginning ought to be made upon a widespread health education campaign centring upon nutrition—ideally, one in which both the agriculturalists and the food industry would become partners and allies with the health professionals. It is heartening to realise that something of this kind has begun to happen: in 1978, for example, four panels of specialists representing agricultural, food industry and health interests were convened for a conference on Food, Health and Farming. Over a period of five months each panel studied those food components considered to be related to health risks, with particular reference to the implications for UK agriculture of any changes in food consumption. In their report, they stated that they had 'identified significant gaps in knowledge, and apparent conflicts between the manner of food production, the value of the food produced and its consequences for health on consumption'.[4]

Perhaps most of all leaders are needed with real conviction of the necessity for change and the resolution to see this carried out. Such are indeed to be found in Scotland today. Especially noteworthy is the McCarrison Society, of which a strong branch exists north of the Border, bringing together doctors, dentists, nutritionists, farmers, housewives—all in fact who are concerned about the quality of today's diet. They are committed to the teaching of pioneer doctor/nutritionist Sir Robert McCarrison (mentioned in an earlier chapter) that for positive health man requires a varied, nutritious diet of whole foods grown on fertile soil.

The President of the Society is a Scot, Dr Walter Yellowlees, a doughty fighter over many years for a more wholesome diet in Scotland. He takes a depressed view of today's health picture. In the James Mackenzie Lecture to the Royal College of Practitioners in 1978 he said:

> I believe it to be true that in those countries which have achieved unparalleled advance in technological skill in medicine and in what is called standard of living we are witnessing the decay of man—the decay of his teeth, his arteries, his bowels and his joints on a colossal and unprecedented scale.[5]

Clearly he views the mounting toll of ill-health with deep concern—not least, the alarming incidence of malignant disease with, as he stresses, 'a heavy preponderance of bowel cancer'. One might be forgiven for imagining that he is making these gloomy observations somewhere, say, in the middle of Glasgow. Not so: he is talking of rural Perthshire. And bearing in mind the comparatively stress-free and open-air lifestyle of many of his patients (not to mention the great contrast between their health record and that of their forebears as described in the old *Statistical Account* some 200 years ago) it is perhaps small wonder that he has little hesitation in laying the major part of the blame at the door of a single environmental factor—diet. He affirms:

> It cannot be shouted from the rooftops often enough or loud enough that unless first priority is given to nutrition, health education will always be ineffective and will fail. No matter how much exercise we take, how good our houses; no matter if we are non-smokers, are free of stress and spend regular hours standing on our heads or contemplating our own umbilicus, if our food is not right, we will not have health.

10

WORLD HUNGER

Should this affect the way we eat?

One would hope that by this time a reasonable case had been made for modifying our food habits in Scotland for the sake of our health. But could there be any other reasons for changing the way we eat? I believe that there is another reason and that it is a very powerful one. It is simply this, that there are in the world today something around one thousand million people who are, according to the most recent set of World Bank figures, either starving to death or 'living in a state of permanent and crippling poverty'.

What has the food—or lack of food—of the poor world got to do with how we eat here in Scotland? A very great deal. Two main reasons come immediately to mind. In the first place, many of the statistics of starvation are only too well known to us. Not simply statistics either, but people—men, women and, perhaps especially, children, who through the medium of television come right into our livingrooms, bringing their desperate plight with them. The late Lord Ritchie Calder put it thus in 1962:

> Today, the world has shrunk in space and time. In terms of transport and communications, all countries and all people are neighbours. The child who dies in the Baluba country of the Congo, in the gutters of Calcutta, or the mountains of Bolivia, is as great a reproach to us today as the child who once died of hunger, or the consequences of hunger, on Tyneside or in the valleys of South Wales.[1]

(Or, he might have added, in the tenements of our Scottish cities). Would it not perhaps be true to affirm that our awareness of the hungry today is in a sense greater than was that of the citizens of Edinburgh, say, of the Irish and Highland folk who died in the potato famines of the mid 1840s?

The second reason why I believe world hunger to be totally relevant to us in Scotland is simply that we are part of the developed world, and it is in no small measure due to the way the

144

developed world lives and eats and wastefully uses up resources that the poor of the undeveloped world starve.

Of course there are other reasons—like wars and the astronomical sums expended on armaments, as well as natural disasters and ignorance, not to mention much greed, injustice and oppression within the countries concerned. It seems very clear, however, that the oft-repeated statement that they starve because the world cannot produce enough food is a myth: on the contrary, reliable authorities have calculated that each year ample is produced to feed every man, woman and child on the entire globe: the trouble is that it is gobbled up by those who can afford to pay for it. 'Hunger is not a scourge', wrote Susan George in *How the Other Half Dies*; 'it is a disgrace.'[2]

In the face of such facts, could it be said that we in Scotland have the right to choose our food purely on the basis of what we *like* to eat? I believe very strongly that such an attitude can in no way be justified.

There are certain distinct parallels between the situation worldwide today and that which prevailed in our own country in the past. Hunger was no stranger to a great many of our ancestors. As recently as the 1930s, Sir John (later Lord) Boyd Orr was campaigning on behalf of the poor with crusading zeal. Lord Ritchie Calder wrote of him:

> He was angry and frustrated. He could get neither the people nor the Government interested in the nutrition of children. At that time there was a glut of milk. Skimmed milk was being poured down the drain. He had urged the Government to pour it instead down children's throats.[3]

A problem, surely, with a familiar ring to it. How often it was to recur in later years, as food was dumped, or burned, or stock-piled as 'mountains' in one part of the world while in another part people starved to death. Of course there are no easy answers to this appalling problem. Not only do hungry folk not necessarily welcome unfamiliar food: it is obviously a question of economics. Farmers must be paid for what they produce. In 1973, for example, a time of acute world food shortage and widespread famine, the US Government was actually paying farmers to keep land out of production. The fact that there are no easy answers, however, need not mean that no way forward can possibly be found.

Every decade since the Second World War has had its own special initiative to end hunger. In the 1940s it was largely out of Lord Boyd Orr's vision that the Food and Agricultural Organisation of the United Nations (whose first Director-General he became) came into existence, one of its aims being 'to improve the nutrition of the peoples of all countries'. In 1960, it was the Freedom from Hunger Campaign. In the 1970s—an era of serious world food shortages—the World Food Council was established following the Third World Food Conference held in Rome in 1974. Yet the realisation of its stated aims, 'that within a decade no child will go to bed hungry, no family will fear for its next day's bread and no human being's future will be stunted by malnutrition', today seems further off than ever.

As the decade of the 1980s was opening, people everywhere were beginning to read the Brandt Report,[4] in which an international Commission under the chairmanship of West German Chancellor Willi Brandt proclaimed that 'there must be an end to mass hunger and malnutrition'; urged determined international co-operation, and made the grim prediction: 'There is a real danger that in the year 2000 a large part of the world's population will still be living in poverty.' And finally, as recently as October 1981 the much-publicised Mexico Summit—which met in a purpose-built ultra-luxury resort to look for solutions to world poverty and hunger—turned out a dismal failure. Why? It is difficult to avoid the conclusion that it was because of the rich nations' refusal to yield an inch to the demands of the poor countries that those policies which perpetuate the ever-widening gap between haves and have-nots be changed.

Consider a few of the facts. In the rich industrial sector of the world, some 25 per cent of the global population consumes well over 50 per cent of the world's food, uses up around 85 per cent of its energy and some 80 per cent of its fertilisers—and in addition controls the world market which fixes the prices the poor world will receive for its primary products. At the same time more than 90 per cent of the world's scientists and technologists are working to improve the living conditions of that same 25 per cent of the global population.

Meanwhile, in the poor world, an estimated 10,000 people die each day from the effects of malnutrition; one child in four dies before its first birthday, and of those who do survive, many suffer irreversible brain damage due to protein malnutrition in early child-hood. An estimated 35 per cent to 50 per cent of all mankind lives without access to health services of any kind. And each year huge numbers of children go blind because of simple lack of one nutri-ent—vitamin A. This must surely be a challenging thought to all of us who have an interest in food and nutrition.

In the context of this study, only the briefest look at the world
food situation is possible: there is an obvious risk of over-general-
isation or simplification. But, inasmuch as potential changes in our
own food habits are involved, the risk has to be taken. Take just
one vital food staple, grain. Because of the pressing need to earn
foreign currency, cereals are regularly *exported* from countries in
which much of the population is under-fed or even starving. Where
does it go? To the developed world, where the bulk of it will be fed
not directly to humans but instead 'through' cattle, poultry and
pigs, to be eaten eventually in the form of those animal protein
foods on which we have become accustomed to basing our meals.
That this is a wasteful process most are probably now aware: it
takes several pounds of grain to produce a single pound of meat. It
is reckoned, in fact, that animals (including pets) in the developed
world consume more grain than the entire population of India and
China added together.

One who had much to say about the root causes of deprivation
and poverty was the late Dr E F Schumacher, economist and author
of *Small is Beautiful.* The sub-title of his book, *Economics as if
People Mattered,* gives a clue to his thinking.[5] First, he saw clearly
that wherever there is callous disregard for people, wherever greed
comes before human need, misery and disaster are, in the long run,
inevitable. This process can take many forms—like encouraging
dangerous dependence on 'cash crop' monoculture at the expense
of food production, or reserving vast tracts of prime land for
rearing beef cattle. More recently, the totally inappropriate pushing
of baby milk sales in poor countries provided a particularly distressing example.

Schumacher's answers to world problems cut across much of the
accepted thinking of his time, but the principles he laid down
underlie much of the development work of the caring aid agencies.
He saw that people in poor countries share a vital need with all
people everywhere, the need to work; they need above all to be
taught how to help themselves—'not a handout, but a hand up', as
someone has put it. Instead of aid being channelled via huge,
prestigious urban projects employing western-type technology—
which can actually exacerbate local problems—it must reach the
poor who desperately need it. Schumacher therefore advocated
'appropriate technology', the gentle alternative, coming 'somewhere between the combine-harvester and the sickle', so that
human labour is supplemented, not displaced, by machines. Along
these lines, then, have come into being hundreds of small, predominantly rural self-help schemes designed to check the drift of people

to the cities in search of work and food, and to allow rural folk to find their own level of development in appropriate, practical ways.

Tear Fund's director, Rev George Hoffman—deeply involved over many years in development issues—recently said:

> We have seen that the superimposing of a Western pattern of technology and Western techniques on a developing community is a blueprint for failure. We have learned, and are still learning, to listen. And to listen again. To listen to others who have made mistakes. To listen to the local leaders and elders. And, after listening, to be ready to modify, adjust and adapt in order that the real source of a community's problems will be tackled instead of just treating the symptoms.[6]

Which is in accord with Schumacher's belief:

> As long as we think we know, when in fact we do not, we shall continue to go to the poor and demonstrate to them all the marvellous things they could do if they were already rich.

Both, indeed, have stressed the need to *improve* traditional methods (rather than to sweep them away), thus making possible more and better local production; and breaking the well-known vicious circle of inadequate food leading to disease and lack of energy, leading to lowered food production, leading to inadequate food supply.

Inadequate food—which is where this discussion began. What, if anything, can we do to alleviate world hunger and misery? Or are the numbers involved so vast, is the problem so hopeless, that nothing will possibly help? Suppose we were seriously to follow out the now-familiar slogan coined by one of the development agencies and 'live simply that others may simply live', what effect would this be likely to have? Would they, in fact, have an appreciably greater chance of survival? What lifestyle changes would be envisaged— with special reference to food? The crucial question was touched upon earlier, i.e. that millions of tons of grain needed by the poorer countries are imported by the developed world to be fed 'through' livestock to produce meat. It is essentially meat production, then, which has to be looked at in the light of world needs. More particularly, it is beef—and to a lesser extent poultry and pigs: sheep feed on grassland, often on hilly areas not suitable for other purposes. There are in the world many kinds of crop residues suitable for animal feeding—not to mention grass. Granted that we in this country are less guilty in this respect than, for example, the USA,

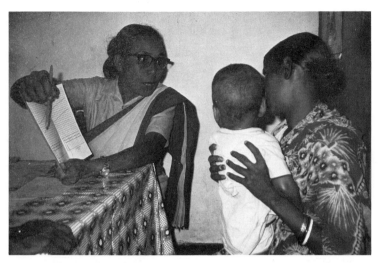

16a Under 5's clinic—the health worker explains to the mother that the weight of her child is just below the safe levels of the 'Road to Health chart'. *Source* **Tear Fund**

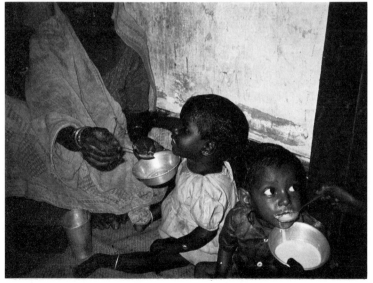

16b A nutritional rehabilitation centre in a refugee camp in Dacca, Bangladesh. Teaching mothers to spoonfeed children with appropriate and available foods. *Source* **Tear Fund**

can it be seen as justifiable to feed animals on grain fit for human consumption while elsewhere human beings are starving to death? An article in the *British Medical Journal* in the late 1970s said:

> Western-type diet with its high meat content leads to an extremely inefficient use of land and food resources. A switch to a more vegetarian-type diet would enable enough grains and vegetables to be grown to provide sustenance for every person on earth. Apart from personal example, which is having an effect, a change in diet and the pattern of agriculture could be achieved through a national programme to educate people on the health benefits of eating less meat and animal fat, and an overhaul of Government aid to farmers to discourage meat production.[7]

Another article in the same journal called for a move away from our 'steakhouse mentality'. The above sentence about Government aid to farmers is clearly important, illustrating as it does the fact that every policy change of this sort always involves somebody's living, so reasonable alternatives as well as compensation have to be thought through with some urgency.

What might 'a switch to a more vegetarian-type diet' mean in practical terms? Many responsible people have in recent years become vegetarians for this kind of reason. Most of us would not perhaps feel impelled to do so (or would believe that livestock are an integral part of the ecological environment), but it could mean each family having, say, a couple of meatless days per week, or possibly concentrating on the kind of main meal in which a small amount of meat is eked out by vegetables, cereals, potatoes, pulses. This theme will be further developed in the next chapter.

Can we somehow, however gradually, begin by eliminating the deeply-ingrained idea that all our main meals must be built around meat? Recently on radio the wife of an unemployed industrial worker, when asked about the dinners she now gave her family, replied: 'Nowadays we can never afford anything but mince and sausages.' But there is a whole range of excellent vegetarian dishes, or dishes using minimal meat or fish, which would cost far less. And when we do have vegetarian dishes on the menu, must they masquerade as cutlets and roasts rather than being served, so to speak, in their own right?

Let us note a few of the new protein sources, conventional and unconventional, which may well come to form a greater part of our future food. It is possible to produce protein food from lowly organisms (such as bacteria, yeasts and fungi) which grow with great rapidity. Algae too can be cultured to produce food—

although probably for animals rather than humans on account of the cost of extraction involved. Organisms can even be grown on hydrocarbon residues ('oil protein'). Leaf protein in the form of pressed cakes has been tried out extensively in needy areas, admittedly with rather varied degrees of success. In all of this, one aspect has claimed much attention: in order to become a useful source of food for humans, all types of unconventional food must have an acceptable taste—and smell—since unfortunately people sometimes prefer to starve rather than eat what is strange and unpalatable.

Soya, a pulse which has been used in China for some 5,000 years, is well recognised as one of the world's most economical protein sources: it is estimated that a single acre of this crop can produce enough protein to meet the needs of one person for as much as six years. It is already quite widely used as a filler in products such as pies and sausage rolls: also because we tend to dislike mushy foods, various types of meatless meats have been prepared by a process of spinning, mainly from soya and groundnuts, so as to give a texture resembling that of meat. The fact that the residues from these crops make good fodder for livestock is obviously another point in their favour.

Although much work has been done in recent years on producing various fish concentrates, it cannot yet be claimed that a truly acceptable product for human use has been perfected. On the conventional side, however, fish farming is proving a success in many parts of the world, including Scotland, and provided prices can be brought within an attainable range, these cultivated fish could provide a welcome addition to our diet. Fish production throughout the world could indeed show a colossal upward swing: experiments in the USA and Japan, for instance, have demonstrated that mussels grown attached to strings suspended in water can give immense yields.

There is, finally, one particular aspect of world food supplies and meat-eating which concerns me as a dietitian a great deal. It is that, because of the high incidence of overweight and obesity in the developed world, an ever-growing number of people are being advised to follow diets based to a large extent on meat and fish and using a minimal amount of cereals. This is precisely the kind of dietary advice I used to give in the past, and which I regret in the light of present knowledge, believing strongly that such regimes should be used only in the initial phase of reducing weight, if at all.

Supposing, then, that we in Scotland were to make substantial changes in our food habits, or even that many millions throughout the developed world were to do so, can it be said that this would really relieve world hunger? So far as I can at present ascertain, while it would emphatically represent an important step in the right direction, especially if taken in conjunction with the elimination of all wasteful forms of human and animal feeding, to suggest that it would solve overnight such a colossal global problem would be naive and misleading. As things stand, since the problem is vastly more complex than a simple matter of redistribution, it could even result merely in less grain being grown. Really effective action to eliminate world hunger and poverty would require to go much further and deeper. It would demand decisive action by world authorities to bring about profound changes in, for example, land ownership, the practices of the multinational trading companies and, most of all, international trading structures.

While most of the health problems of the poorer nations stem from deprivation and undernutrition, most of our own have their origin in excess. If it can be shown that a more simple and economical mode of eating—using, for instance, fewer meat foods and fats, and more cereals and vegetables—would in fact not only benefit the poor nations but also lead to improvements in our own health, could there be any cogent reason for delaying these changes? Would not we, were the situations reversed and we were the hungry, expect just such action on our behalf?

In recent years many experts have come to believe that the world's food problems can be solved only by a global approach. In an address to the 1981 international conference in Paris, entitled 'Towards a Global Approach to Food and Agriculture', Claude Aubert, an agricultural adviser with an unsurpassed knowledge of world food problems, finished thus:

> I will end by once more repeating what is too often forgotten: that technical solutions to the problems of the Third World are known and that their application is not particularly difficult. Successful application, however, depends both in the industrialised countries and in the countries of the Third World, on the political will to encourage a different type of development and a more equitable division of resources.[8]

11

SCOTLAND'S FUTURE DIET

Where do we go from here?

What makes people eat the way they do? This is a fascinating subject—worthy of a study by itself, and more worthy of a sociologist
than a dietitian—but one at which we shall take a brief look. First
and foremost, probably, should be noted such factors as habit,
family traditions and simple availability of foods. Writing on this,
Professor John Hawthorn, of Strathclyde University, points out:
'That splendid biological variability which decrees the difference
between the Scot and the Hottentot, the Spaniard and the Chinese
. . . decrees also that one man's meat is another man's poison'.[1]
Who could easily imagine Scots, even extremely hungry Scots,
falling with relish upon the traditional Papua New Guinean feasts
of toasted beetle-grubs, any more than Papua New Guineans
showing immediate acceptance of haggis, tatties and neeps?

Price in relation to income is clearly a potent factor in determining food choice. There must be many large families, for
instance, whose preference might well be for butter, but who will
choose margarine because it is cheaper and goes further. Nowadays, too, attractive appearance of food—whether real or as
advertised by the media—obviously plays a major part: some
housewives have in fact confided to interviewers that they seldom
or never make a list, preferring to pick up whatever takes their
fancy in their journey round the supermarket. Ease of preparation,
too, will certainly decree preference in a great many cases: no
wonder that the advertising term 'fast food' finds so much favour
nowadays. In Scotland, food preferences based on religious beliefs
play a fairly minor role—except in the case of the small Asian
population—although the number of vegetarian diets, based for
example on Zen Buddhism, has grown in recent years. What we
used to call 'food fads and fallacies' (the kind of belief typified by
'brown eggs are more nourishing than white') are still, I believe,
pretty widespread in Scotland. The growing demand for health

foods we looked at earlier, in Chapter 5. What about actual
nutritional knowledge? One would like to think that for a reasonable number of Scots housewives, mainly perhaps those younger
ones who have studied the subject at school, this does play a significant part, although claims that certain foods have slimming proper-
ties probably have a far wider influence.

One interesting factor remains to be mentioned. It is that food is,
unfortunately, subject to prestige value—in other words snobbery.
One might be tempted to think that this is a fairly recent phenom-
enon, but one would be wrong. Looking at the history of bread, we
saw (Chapter 6) that all down the ages white bread had far higher
prestige than the darker-coloured variety. Now the time may have
arrived when it becomes socially unacceptable to serve anything but
wholemeal. Similarly with barley a see-saw effect can be observed:
it fell in the social scale from the late eighteenth century onwards,
but is now enjoying a modest resurgence as a health food. Tea
when it first appeared was a very snobbish—and of course expensive—beverage: now it is probably considered somewhat more
humble than coffee. And take the case of vegetables—is it not true
that the smart hostess generally prefers to serve courgettes at her
winter dinner-party, rather than the excellent—and arguably,
superior—leeks growing in her own garden?

All the above factors, and doubtless several more, would have to
be borne in mind supposing that, in the face of mounting evidence
and concern about the health issues we have been considering, the
powers-that-be were eventually to be convinced of the need to
tackle ill-health from the angle of prevention, and to mount a
nationwide campaign to raise levels of nutrition. Obviously special
needs would have to be taken into account—whether of elderly
people, immigrants, food faddists or whatever—while, as has been
pointed out earlier, it would be necessary to secure the help of the
food industry both as regards actual products and in their advertising of these. Speaking recently on radio, Mr Denis Burkitt, a
surgeon and a leading protagonist for increasing the cereal fibre
content of our diet, said that in response to demand there has
already been a 'slight but positive response' from the food
industry—for example, cereal products with higher fibre content
being introduced. He went on to say that the industry has always
maintained that its products are aimed at supplying popular
demand. So any nutrition campaign must aim to change and
improve the quality of what the public demands. That any such
campaign would have to be a fairly mammoth operation and cost a
great deal cannot be denied. Yet expenditure on preventive

medicine, including nutrition education, is at present a mere fraction of what is spent on health repairs. And, while no absolutely immediate returns could be expected, it could be argued that the long-term savings in medical care would be very considerable indeed.

Who exactly would be taught, and by what means? The simple answer would be that ideally every age group from the beginning of life to the end should be reached and influenced. The importance of good nutrition during pregnancy has in fact long been recognised: many dietitians too would doubtless agree that one can teach nutrition to no more highly motivated group, particularly those expecting their first child. But more recent research has shown that this emphasis does not begin early enough. Much evidence exists to show that poor nutrition can play a significant part in causing, for example, stillbirths and neonatal deaths: the first few weeks after conception are vital in fetal development. It cannot therefore be stressed too strongly that the right time to ensure a woman's nutritional status is before pregnancy begins at all.

Included in this area of teaching would be an emphasis on breast-feeding as the ideal (although, since not every mother is able to achieve this, such teaching must always be approached sensitively, healthy alternative feeding methods being taught as well). Next would come the teaching of basic principles of nutrition to mothers of toddlers and young children, and indeed to women—and if possible, men—of all age-groups, including for example those preparing for retirement.

Imaginative projects centring on food and health could also play a greater part in the pursuits of the various youth organisations. But it need hardly be said that schools should be made a real focus of nutrition education, something which is in fact happening to a greater extent nowadays. Nor should such teaching be confined either to girls or to those specifically studying home economics. A strong plea for food education to be made really practical was made recently by Alan Harrison in the journal *Nutrition and Food Science*. In an article entitled *Food Education and School Meals: Are They on Separate Tables?* he points out the anomalies which can often exist between theoretical food education in the classroom and some of the actual food choices confronting pupils in school meals, not to mention school tuckshops. He urges determined moves towards an integrated plan, encompassing not only good nutrition but also the social aspects of eating, and, in the face of mounting consumer pressures, teaching pupils to make personal evaluations of foods.[2]

Finally, there would ideally be far more emphasis on nutrition in the curricula of all those involved in health care, from the medical and nursing professions all the way through to those with less obvious, but still important, responsibilities for the health of large numbers of people. An obvious example in this category would be the large corps of home helps, through whom one might hope to improve nutritional standards among our huge and ever-growing geriatric population. But the long-established food habits of this last group are not by any means easily influenced—and certainly not by a mere set of lectures.

Supposing then that this hypothetical mass campaign in nutrition education had actually been carried out, would it be likely that everyone had been reached? Unfortunately not. Whether one is thinking of youth organisations or women's groups, or even of mothers attending an antenatal clinic, would it not be true to say that it is always the well-motivated who take the trouble to attend? And yet the real object is to make an impact on the others.

How might this be accomplished? It is possible that a really practical, down-to-earth teaching series on television, using carefully chosen illustrations, would be very helpful. A more personal approach, if this could somehow be managed, would almost certainly accomplish far more. Perhaps the scheme which has proved so successful in the campaign for adult literacy might be a good model to follow: some women—born housewives, budget-planners, cooks—might well be happy to pass on their skills in a really practical way to less able fellow-housewives.

Here we could well have a valuable lesson to learn from the undeveloped world where, in some areas, health aides—chosen by the community itself, not for educational attainments but for wisdom, character and personality—are trained in basic health care and then proceed to pass on their acquired knowledge and skills to others—by all accounts, with a remarkable degree of success. In a few instances community nutrition workers have in fact been recruited in the UK but not, to my knowledge, in Scotland. The idea has certainly much to recommend it, since not only would cultural barriers be eliminated, but there are simply not sufficient professionally-trained personnel to undertake, on such a scale, teaching which would have to include, as well as nutrition, the basic principles of good housekeeping, budgeting, menu-planning and cookery.

The more informal this teaching could be made, and the more it could be brought into the specific local situation (possibly with the help of a Health Committee recruited from the community) the better. The aim of such teaching would of course be not simply to pass on knowledge for its own sake, but actually to *change behaviour.* In the typically restrained language of officialdom, the following statement is made in the report, *National Food Policy in the UK:*[3] 'There is a gap between the possession of knowledge and its application in practice.' In more homely terms—teach nutrition to your heart's content, but try to see at the end of it all what people are actually putting into their baskets when they go shopping.

Who should be responsible for planning and administering such a national campaign of nutrition education? The extent to which Government should dictate what we eat is a matter of debate in this country. We do not at present have a national food and nutrition policy to the extent, say, that Canada and the USA or the Scandinavian countries do. Government is, of course, responsible generally for ensuring that the food supply is safe and wholesome, and for allocating food subsidies, as well as, on the specifically nutritional side, for such measures as the fortification of the popular staples bread and margarine, and making available certain supplements to children at risk of undernutrition. However, particularly in view of current concern over the diseases of affluence, many people believe strongly that Government should adopt a much more specific, positive role, ensuring that it is the healthiest foods which are the cheapest. Others believe just as strongly that a too-aggressive dictation by the State of the way we eat would represent a real infringement of individual liberty. The debate continues.

By what means do we actually know how people are eating at any given time? Various dietary surveys, usually on a small scale, are carried out as part of a routine research programme. For an overall view of food consumption trends, however, we depend largely upon the National Food Survey which has been undertaken annually ever since 1940. Each year a sample cross-section of the community, comprising some 7,000 households or around 20,000 people, is selected, the housewives chosen supplying information on the type and quantity of food they buy. Since extras like alcohol and sweets are not included, figures for these are supplied respectively by HM Customs and Excise and the Cocoa, Chocolate and Confectionery Alliance. All of this information, while undeniably of immense value, does have its limitations—in particular in that while family intakes are known, those of individuals are not.

Out of several trends which these statistics show, only the outstanding ones need to be mentioned here. There has been since the war a marked increase in fat consumption. At the end of the war fat supplied some 30 per cent of the energy in the British diet: now it has risen to over 40 per cent. Also, from the mid 1950s alcohol has shown a significant upward trend, the rise having become steeper since around 1970. We observed earlier, too, that the pattern in increasing affluence is that sugar tends to displace starchy foods—which can at the same time mean a reduction in fibre content—and that this has happened in the UK. Finally, the common tendency to increase energy intake without increasing energy expenditure has been followed in this country.

In view of all this, many experts in recent years have offered guidelines towards a 'prudent diet'. In 1978, for instance, the booklet *Eating for Health* was published by the Department of Health and Social Security.[4] Miss Dorothy Hollingsworth, quoted earlier, has recommended that in the face of today's serious health problems and our current dietary habits, we must find a diet which contains less fat than we have been accustomed to eating for some years; increase the starchy cereal and vegetable foods in our diet, as well as using smaller proportions of 'empty calorie' foods, i.e. sugar, some fats and alcohol. She then adds, very wisely, that this must at the same time be 'a diet which accommodates personal preferences and in no way detracts from the pleasure of eating'.

The pleasure of eating—yes, indeed. This seems to me to be of paramount importance when it comes to Scotland's food. There are several things which I strongly believe those of us who want to see improvement in the Scottish diet must bear in mind if we are to tackle the problem in a sensible and practical manner. We must at all costs shed the crank image, with its overtones of gritting one's teeth and swallowing rather unattractive food rather as one would pills. We must dispel the notion that a healthy diet necessarily involves paying a lot of money for something esoteric called health food; and we must somehow put across to the public that there are many simple—and indeed downright economical—ways of building upon and improving our own traditional diet, rather than changing it out of all recognition, and even leaving it recognisably Scottish at the end.

What is the best way to teach nutrition? Clearly there are a whole variety of ways in which information may be presented, depending of course upon the type of audience and the time available. In my young days as a dietitian, we felt it incumbent upon us, no matter *what* the occasion, to wade doggedly through every single one of the nutrients—protein, fat, carbohydrate, minerals, vitamins, water, roughage, the lot—sending our unfortunate audience away, no doubt, in a kind of bemused fog of orange juice and sunshine and carrots and wholemeal bread and carbohydrate and liver and protein: no wonder we were seldom invited back! Nowadays, thankfully, the approach is altogether simpler and, unless in the case of a whole teaching series in depth, people will be taught (with the help of a wide range of imaginative audio-visual aids) about *foods* rather than nutrients, and assisted to choose a healthy diet tailored to suit their individual requirements. It will be emphasised that a diet implies essentially a mixture of foods, and that in fact satisfactory mixtures may be obtained from a wide variety of sources—variety, indeed, being an extremely important factor.

We have looked at Scotland's health problems and her most glaring (general) dietary faults—too many foods containing sugar and refined starch; too many fats, including too much fried food; too many of the inferior type of processed foods; lack of fresh and fibrous foods; in some cases, too much of everything. At the same time we have noted the experts' recommendations for a prudent diet—to cut back on sugar, fats and alcohol, and to step up consumption of whole cereals, vegetables and fruit; and, in view of the global food crisis, the responsibility of those in the richer sector to cut back on meat foods.

One dietary constituent which we have not mentioned is salt. Food experts have during the past few decades changed their minds—and changed them back again—about whether or not high intakes are linked with hypertension (high blood pressure). Today, a great deal of research would certainly seem to show that they are. What of intakes in Scotland? These might generally tend to be high, even as regards that most heinous of crimes—sprinkling salt on untasted soup! But although experts are generally agreed that less salt should be used both in cooking and at table, advice on this is not at all straightforward; and many who do not use much salt at table might, for example, find they have a high intake because of a fondness for preserved foods such as kippers, cheese, bacon and tinned meats or fish. Some processed snacks, too, have a high salt content.

Now for the crucial question. What, in the light of all these considerations, *is* the sort of 'food mixture' which could be recommended as the best for Scots to choose their diet from today? This is surely the point at which one must take a deep breath, state one's firm beliefs and be ready to defend them. This, too, is the point at which we should take serious note of the lessons our own history has to teach.

From a study of the vagaries of our ancestors' diet, one thing emerges clearly—or so it seems to me. It is that by far the best period was that following the agricultural improvements of the late eighteenth century, a dietary era (Chapter 3) which continued in some rural areas right up to the first two decades of this century. At that time the principal components were oats and barley, dairy foods and eggs, potatoes and a (limited) number of other vege- tables and wild plants, a variable and often generous supply of fish, depending on area, and meat occasionally or in smallish amounts—the quantity of this generally increasing during the nine- teenth century. We should at the same time recall the usually highly favourable impressions of the health and physique of those same rural folk recorded both by visitors to Scotland and by the resident writers, for example in the *Statistical Account*.

In widely different parts of the world researchers have identified diets of quite remarkable similarity to this one as producing out- standingly healthy people. The Hunza tribe in the Himalayan foot- hills, for example, were found by Sir Robert McCarrison to enjoy excellent health and unusual longevity. In seven years of careful observation, no single case of heart disease, cancer, diabetes, peptic ulcer, multiple sclerosis, or appendicitis was diagnosed among them. And their diet? Practically a replica of that of our ancestors quoted above, except that—not altogether surprisingly—it scored higher marks for fruit and vegetables. It comprised principally whole wheat, maize and barley; milk and butter; a variety of fruits, vegetables and pulses; meat on special occasions only. Both the Scottish and the Indian example typify a diet based essentially upon whole, as opposed to refined, cereal grains and dairy foods—two groups which are recognised as forming excellent supplements to each other—with other, mainly plant, foods making up for the nutrients which they lack. It should not, however, be forgotten that in the coastal areas of Scotland fish was a very important constitu- ent.

Undoubtedly the nearest Scotland has approached to this kind of diet in fairly recent times was during the Second World War, with its rationing of such items as sugar and sweets, fats and meat, and heavy emphasis on potatoes, green vegetables, pulses and cereals. Soon after it had ended, Scots nutrition expert Dr (later Professor) R Passmore was able to make the arresting statement: 'Probably never before in history, and certainly not in living memory, have the children of Scotland been so healthy.'[5]

Would it not therefore seem like good sense to base our diet at least to some extent on the traditional pattern, modifying it of course to include the far greater variety which modern palates demand, as well as rectifying the ancient failing—lack of vegetables and fruit?

Here is a tentative outline of what I have in mind:

Begin with porridge or muesli for breakfast, adding fruit or fruit juice as often as possible, as well as toast or rolls which, it need hardly be said, should preferably be wholemeal.

For lunch, whether at home or eaten out, a very simple but nutritious meal, such as lentil soup, or Scotch broth (indeed any soup designed as a 'meal in itself') or else baked beans on toast, baked potato with cheese filling, or whenever possible a simple seasonal salad including a protein source such as an egg, some cheese or sardines, with—according to taste and requirement—a wholemeal roll or bread or fruit or yoghurt, and accompanied by milk or fresh fruit or juice. I should like to see many more restaurants serving just this type of lunch.

For dinner or supper, I suggest a main dish which on some days could be vegetarian, and which on others could incorporate a *small* amount of meat or fish filled out with such starchy ingredients as potatoes, oatmeal, brown rice or pasta, pulses, cheese pastry—the kind of dish, in fact, of which every country can provide excellent samples—all the way from kedgeree and pilau and vegetable/meat curry through quiche lorraine and risotto and spaghetti bolognese to, nearer home, Irish stew and Scottish haggis or stovies. All of these to be served, needless to say, with plentiful helpings of vegetables. For the second course, either yoghurt or fresh or stewed fruit, or occasional puddings with fruit, such as pies or crumbles.

These are obviously merely outlines of the main meals, making no mention either of such extras as butter or margarine or preserves, or of something else dear to Scottish hearts—snacks. These should ideally be of good quality, with emphasis falling on (non-sugary) drinks, or fruit, rather than on sweet things; the guide here being body weight rather than appetite. Whether or not the dentists would agree, I believe that, in this and all other cases, there is room for treats. And what about baking? Again this is something which rates very high in Scotland, good bakers usually being esteemed—at least among older housewives—rather more highly than good cooks. The best answer seems to me to be a determined move towards *plain* baking, using nourishing ingredients—dried fruit, cocoa, treacle, wholemeal flour, oatmeal, rolled oats—so that oatcakes and scones become the norm again. And leave the iced cakes and meringues for parties! One group who do certainly need snacks, on account of their very high energy requirements, are fast-growing adolescents: better that they should eat this kind of snack, at least some of the time, than the junk foods which are customary for so many.

An eating plan of the sort sketched out above should not, one hopes, seem too strange or daunting. It does embody considerable change, however, especially perhaps in the move away from the deeply-ingrained pattern of soup, meat-and-two-veg, pudding type of dinner. It is possible, too, that having no bacon or sausage for breakfast—not so much as an egg to go to work on—and only soup and a roll for lunch might seem like real deprivation to some.

Change will come about only gradually—that is certain. Especially among older Scots housewives, there is suspicion of anything to do with whole or health foods. I have had many questions asked on this subject; such as: 'Doesn't it mean eating a lot of nuts?' Nuts, apart perhaps from peanuts, are traditionally something you eat only very occasionally, or more often hand out to the guisers at Hallowe'en. Another common question is: 'Don't you have to have all your vegetables raw?' In many cases, say with vegetables like carrots or celery, this would certainly be a good idea, and indeed one would greatly like to see more—and much more imaginative—salads gracing the Scottish table, especially in winter; but perhaps more important is a general improvement in the method of cooking those vegetables most commonly used here, such as cabbage, cauliflower and brussels sprouts. Probably our greatest fault in Scotland is over-cooking.

For many, though, the greatest barrier comes at the mention of wholemeal flour—above all, stoneground wholemeal flour. But a growing number of women in Scotland today, and of men also, have learned to bake their own wholemeal bread. Those who at present use nothing but the inevitable white and refined might begin a gradual move away from this by trying out the browner flours, or even adding some bran to their scones, pastry or shortbread—and then comparing the results: it is at least possible that they would find their taste had changed. Even better, perhaps, would be an all-out campaign to increase substantially the use of our excellent traditional cereal, oats—not only in porridge, muesli and oatcakes, but also using oatmeal and rolled oats in biscuits, gingerbread and fruit crumbles, or as a thickener in soups.

The interesting thing is that oatmeal consumption in Scotland seems likely to receive an unexpected boost. In the autumn of 1981, a report from the USA hit the headlines with the news that an American doctor had identified a miracle food which had the effect of regulating both sugar and fats in blood, and which was being recommended in the treatment of diabetes, heart disease and hypertension. The miracle food was none other than oatmeal porridge. At roughly the same time, a report from North East Scotland told

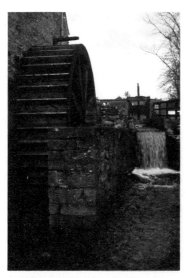

17a   Exterior of Working Oats Mill, Blair Atholl. Photograph Rev
       George Thomson, 1984

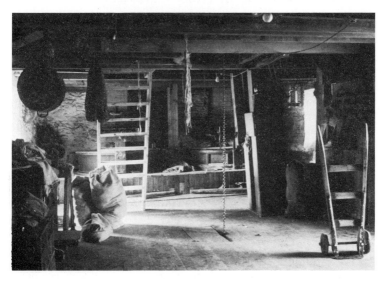

17b   Interior of Working Oats Mill, Mill of Newmill, Auchterless. Sack-
       barrow in foreground, chain and trap-door for sack-hoist in centre,
       grindstones in background. Photograph Alexander Fenton, 1962

the heartening news of increased profits (and even of a meal mill previously threatened with closure given a new lease of life), because of an upward trend in oatmeal consumption. All of this had come about largely because of the popularity of a breakfast product containing oat flakes and bran. Surely it would be a welcome sight to see the old meal mills grinding again in the Scottish glens, instead of serving as museums.

To return, however, to the suggested eating plan outlined above. What of its nutritional value?

To illustrate this a little more clearly, there are set out below three examples from a wide potential range of (winter) menus, alongside an example of the more conventional menu to be found in common use in Scotland today. For ease of discussion, I have called the new plan A and the old B.

Calculation of the nutritional value of menus such as these, allowing for average servings, shows Type A to be well-balanced and to have a marked overall superiority over Type B. A few points are of particular interest. Recent research has linked carotene— found in coloured and green vegetables (especially carrots) and certain fruits, and converted in the body to vitamin A—with protection against some forms of cancer: thus inclusion of these is now seen by some experts as very important. Totals for vitamins of the B group and for vitamin C are good: to ensure winter intake of vitamin D a recommended concentrate taken occasionally might be advisable, especially for children and the elderly—bearing in mind, however, that it is potentially dangerous to take too much of this particular vitamin. As meats have the highest iron content, it might also be as well to remember that alternative sources are eggs, pulses, dried fruits, treacle, cocoa and whole cereals.

What about protein? In a low meat diet it is this nutrient, required for body-building, which gives rise to most queries. Calculation of Type A menus reveals that totals are around 55 to 60 g, giving a safe margin above the accepted minimum levels. The main protein sources in these menus are of course dairy foods and eggs, along with fish, wholegrains, pulses and possibly nuts, and small or occasional servings of meat. One pint of milk supplies nearly 20 g; thus when needs are greater, as in pregnancy or adolescence, an intake of 1½ or 2 pints would be preferable. This also ensures the supply of calcium.

While the sugar content of the Type A menus is clearly fairly low, snacks are by no means absent, extras like baking and preserves being included. Even a modest helping of chips could be permitted once in a while. Also, one pint of milk and 1½ oz of

Recommended Menu (Type A)   Conventional (Type B)

Day 1	Day 2	Day 3	Conventional (Type B)
BREAKFAST			
Orange juice Porridge Wholemeal toast Marmalade	Stewed prunes Muesli Toast Marmalade	Porridge Wholemeal roll Honey	Cornflakes Bacon sandwich White bread Marmalade
LUNCH			
Salad (sardines, lettuce, cheese, raw carrot, cress) Wholemeal roll Oatcake & jam	Lentil soup Wholemeal roll Yoghurt Crispbread, honey	Fresh grapefruit Baked potato, cheese filling Oatcakes, jam	Sausage roll Chips White bread, jam Sweet biscuit
DINNER			
Stovies (potatoes, leeks, onions, small amount leftover meat) Egg custard Stewed apricots	Haggis Turnips & carrots Jacket potatoes Rhubarb crumble (using part oatmeal)	Bacon & egg pie Side salad: sliced (tomatoes, peppers, carrots) French dressing Baked apple and cream	Mince Mashed potatoes Peas Apple tart
THROUGHOUT DAY			
Tea, coffee Wholemeal scone, digestive biscuit 1 pint milk Butter/margarine	Tea, Bovril Oat biscuit Pear 1 pint milk Butter/margarine	Tea, coffee Toasted cheese Treacle scone Orange 1 pint milk Butter/margarine	Tea, coffee Shortbread Sweet biscuits Chocolate biscuit Sweets ½ pint milk Butter/margarine

butter or margarine were allowed for in the calculation. While there should thus be no impression at all that this is meant to be a weight-reducing diet, the energy value is just slightly below recommended levels, and it should certainly not cause overweight. The same could hardly be said of Menu B: in it, both carbohydrate and total energy are much too high, while the fat content adds up to almost double that of the Type A menus. Vitamin totals are poor. As for comparative fibre totals, at this stage it may be a little superfluous even to mention these.

So much for a very brief appraisal of the nutritional value of the suggested menus. There are other aspects to consider, for example cost. Can it be justifiable in Type A menus to include occasional luxuries—fresh cream, for example, and lettuce and tomatoes which are dear in winter? In fact, even with these, the new plan turns out on costing to be very considerably cheaper than the conventional menu.

Finally, does not this way of eating mean a great deal of extra time and trouble? Making one's own soups, baking, even preparing salads in winter—all of these may easily be regarded by busy women as expendable chores. Nobody would deny that there is truth in this. But some of the difficulties can be more imaginary than real. For example in making lentil soup, does assembling all the ingredients in a pan and simmering them (which is practically all that is necessary) really require so much more effort than opening a tin? With practice, too, it can almost certainly take less time to turn out a batch of scones than it would to buy them in a shop. There are, of course, exceptions. Many budget meals can take up a disproportionate amount of time, and are to be avoided. Many housewives have learned to cut corners in every conceivable way and still retain economy and food value. The kind of meals I have in mind are essentially simple, elaborate cooking being reserved for special occasions.

A different kind of claim can be made for this kind of cooking—that it is creative and fulfilling. One of the reasons why I am keen to retain home-made preserves as part of our food is not just that I believe (hopefully) that with simple meals one can get away with a certain amount of sugar, but also for the pure delight of making them, and of seeing them ranged in satisfying rows in the larder afterwards. Those of us who are fortunate enough to be able to raid the hedgerows and produce a whole range of preserves and beverages surely have access to a great deal of creative enjoyment. Could it be that as more women begin to experience the pleasure of serving high quality food which they have themselves prepared—

and perhaps also grown—they might see the role of housewife in an altogether different light? (The argument admittedly has another side: recently a mother of five told me she had taken up sculpture in middle life because everything she had previously created had been eaten up within ten minutes!) Yehudi Menuhin, in his auto-biography *Unfinished Journey*, has an interesting comment about creativity:

> The creative, I firmly hold, is the normal human condition, whether displayed in the kitchen, in housekeeping, in violin-housekeeping or in any of a hundred ways. That there is another definition of normality I am well aware, but I combat strenuously the view that equates the normal with that state of bodily and spiritual undernourishment in which most people have to live.[6]

In a society too much geared to consumerism, creativity is by no means the only casualty. In looking back at our country's history, we saw how many aspects of traditional life—not of course all equally valuable—were lost amid the sweeping changes consequent upon the Industrial Revolution. Some are still being eroded. Especially we noted how the wholesome rural diet gradually deteriorated, and the serious effects of that deterioration. My attention was drawn to a much more extreme example of this process during the time a friend spent working on an island in the Pacific. There, vast profits have been obtained by the inhabitants, who own the phosphate-rich land. Their wealth has brought into being an extremely materialistic society. Having abandoned all attempts at agriculture, they spend much of their time eating, drinking and watching video television. Every item of food has to be imported. Over-indulgence has led to serious health problems: obesity affects young children and adolescents to an alarming degree. 'Healthwise', my friend wrote, 'they are the sickest people I have ever seen.'

This is clearly an unusual case, but it is a frightening instance of what can happen when lifestyle—in this particular case through outside influence on a community—is allowed to become geared to excess, while wholesome traditional ways and values are forgotten. It is a danger which can threaten whenever standard of living, rather than the much more important 'quality of life', is made the primary goal.

Today there is concern in Scotland not only about dietary impoverishment but about certain fundamental agricultural changes. Since the 1950s there has come about a gradual replacement of crop rotation by chemical fertilizers, causing disruption to the whole natural ecological balance between man, animals and the soil: the excessive use of nitrates in particular is believed by some authorities to constitute a serious health hazard.

One need only look at what has happened in the USA. Under the heading 'There's no business like agribusiness', Susan George writes: 'Farming (in America) is a highly sophisticated, highly energy-intensive system for transforming one series of industrial products into another series of industrial products which happen to be edible.'[7] What an unacceptable idea to anyone with the least bit of feeling for the land. Under this agribusiness system, a vast number of small family farms have disappeared, giving place to colossal, streamlined corporate farms producing, at the one end, not only food but also tractors, fertilisers, pesticides: and taking care at the other end of packaging and even marketing of their products. At the same time mechanisation is so intensive that fewer and fewer people are actually working on the land.

The extent to which this pattern is being reproduced in Scotland causes much concern to many thinking people. A growing number of people are taking up environmental issues, or pursuing the goal of self-sufficiency, where there is opportunity, or at least growing some of their own food; while the number of small co-operatives for marketing home-grown produce shows hearteningly steady growth—all demonstrating that small is not only beautiful but possible. On this subject, Dr Walter Yellowlees, McCarrison Society President, has written:

> How can we restore in our land pride of place to the small mixed family farm which conserves and enhances fertility and is the most highly productive unit of all? I do not know the answer to that question, but I am sure that in the present state of the world a nation such as ours, which grows only half of its own food and sees more than a million [he was writing in 1978] *of its men standing idle in the city* streets while thousands of acres stand idle in the countryside, is giving an example not of nationhood but lunacy.[8]

What, then, of the future? If beneficial changes in food and health are to be accomplished, much commitment and determination on the part of a great many people will be required. Take the obvious need for greater self-sufficiency in Scotland. Change will come about when enough people are convinced of the need to work towards it—perhaps, too, when it is realised that it is actually more enjoyable. And at the 'small end' it has certainly begun, with garden-share schemes in operation, waste land being used for gardens, swop-shops for home-grown vegetables and an increasing interest in compost-making. A growing number of people, too, are becoming convinced that it really matters for health that agriculture should be based upon a healthy soil and a right ecological balance, and opting for more emphasis on organic farming—with quality rather than quantity as the goal, and on labour-intensive rather than chemical methods; or turning away from intensive farming, even if that should entail paying more for our food. All of the above ideas represent a lifestyle which does violence neither to human beings, animals, plants, nor to the soil itself—something which for me is summed up by the biblical concept of good stewardship of the earth.

In looking back at the ways of our ancestors, we have concentrated mainly on their dietary practices. There are one or two other aspects which deserve special notice. One feature which is widely known—and which has often provided material for burlesque—is the thrift, or indeed active abhorrence of waste, inherent in the character of the Scots. Much less familiar, possibly, is—in the context of their often dire poverty—the unstinting generosity of their hospitality. For the Celtic peoples in particular this amounted to a law: even if an enemy came under your roof, even if the meal in the barrel was dangerously low, what you had was to be shared.

Many of the early travellers in Scotland have testified to this trait. The celebrated traveller Thomas Pennant mentions that while travelling in Ross-shire the party could scarcely pass a farmhouse without the woman of the house sallying forth to invite them to partake of some milk or whey. This excerpt from Martin Martin's *A Description of the Western Isles of Scotland* (1695) sounds somewhat strange in modern ears:

> They [the Hebrideans] are a very charitable and hospitable people, as is anywhere to be found. The great produce of barley draws many strangers to this island, with a design to procure as much grain as they can; which they get of the inhabitants gratis, only for asking, as they do horses, cows, sheep, wool etc. I was told some months before my last arrival there, that there had been ten men in that place at one time to ask corn gratis, and every one of these had some one, some two, and others three attendants; and during their abode there, were all entertained gratis, no one returning empty.[9]

Hand in hand with hospitality seems to have gone a quite remarkable contempt for excess, particularly in the realm of food. In *The Scottish Gael*, published in 1831, James Logan writes:

> The Celts seem to have considered temperance a virtue, being moderate in eating, banishing hunger by plain fare without curious

dressing. This race has ever been noted for their contempt of delicacies, and their ability to bear privations and fatigue. It has been found that the Highlanders are, when surrounded with plenty, more sparing in their diet than others.[10]

In the same vein, another early tourist, Sacheverell, wrote:

> They bound their appetites by their necessities, and their happiness consists, not in having much but in wanting little. There appeared in all their actions a certain generous air of freedom, and contempt for those trifles, luxury and ambition, which we so servilely creep after.

Considerable numbers throughout the world today are beginning to find that simplicity—even a touch of frugality—can bring back something which tends to be lacking in today's lifestyle—a sense of celebration. Amid the climate of excess which characterises so much of our consumer society, the whole idea of 'treats' has been edged out. In *Enough is Enough* John Taylor says:

> We must learn to turn a small treat into a celebration. A small community, modelled loosely on the old monastic pattern, with which I shared Easter 1974, celebrated the festival by sharing two boxes of fudge after lunch, and such was the skill of their simplicity, it generated more honest excitement and fun than any expensive self-indulgence could have done.[11]

A certain amount of self-denial does not necessarily mean a long face. On the contrary, the simpler the everyday diet, the more enjoyable the special occasions.

Would it not be true to say that to have plenty, and yet to make a deliberate choice to live simply, is a true mark of civilised behaviour? It is, hearteningly, beginning to happen here and there in the world today. Norway, a country with a very high *per capita* income, enjoys the distinction of being the first to decide that 'enough is enough'—or to do so to any significant extent. In a movement which has now spread to Sweden and Denmark, many thousands of Norwegians have chosen to turn their backs on their former affluent lifestyle, living instead in a modest way, eating simple food, supporting conservation and actively opposing pollution, and giving generously to aid development in needy parts of the world. These Scandinavians became aware that their excessively affluent way of life was not only threatening their health but was actually robbing them of the pleasure of living. In the English translation of his book *The Future in Our Hands*, which inspired the launching of the movement of the same name, Norwegian Erik Dammann deplores the loss of simple pleasures in these words:

Do we know what we have lost? We have lost the joy of meeting our needs, because we are never without things for very long. We are used to satisfying the most trivial desire the moment it appears. With only the shadow of an appetite we are munching a hot dog, nibbling a bar of chocolate, or opening the refrigerator. Thirsty for a second, and we get a coke, beer or fruit juice. We fill our time with satisfactions which reduce the experience to zero.

And later:

No, we certainly shall not abandon pleasures. We shall find the genuine ones. In order to become people instead of consumers.[12]

Reading comments such as these, one cannot but feel envious that so many in Scandinavia have already found the secrets of an altogether simpler, happier, and healthier—in the broadest sense of the word—way of living. There is much to be learned from their movement. Yet surely there is as much to be learned, too, as we look back across the centuries, to study for a little and recapture the best in the old life-patterns of our Scottish forebears.

REFERENCES

Chapter 1

1 Stuart Piggott and Keith Henderson *Scotland before History* (Nelson 1958)
2 T C Lethbridge *The Painted Men* (Andrew Melrose, London 1954)
3 Jean Froissart *Chronicles* (Visited Scotland during reign of David II)
4 Robert Chambers *Domestic Annals of Scotland* (Edinburgh 1885)
5 John Taylor (1580–1653) *The Pennyless Pilgrimage (London 1618)*
6 Robert Chambers op. cit.
7 Henry G Graham *The Social Life of Scotland in the Eighteenth Century* (Adam and Charles Black, London 1899)
8 James T Calder *Sketch of the Civil and Traditional History of Caithness* (Wick 1887)
9 *Statistical Account* Vol XII North and West Perthshire (Fortingall)
10 A R B Haldane *The Drove Roads of Scotland* (Nelson 1952)
11 Chamberlayne (visited Scotland 1708)
12 Captain Edward Burt *Letters from a Gentleman in the North of Scotland* (London 1754)
13 Henry G Graham op. cit.
14 Henry G Graham op. cit.
15 *Statistical Account* Vol VII Lanarkshire and Renfrewshire (East Kilbride)
16 *Statistical Account* Vol VII Lanarkshire and Renfrewshire (Cambuslang)

Chapter 2

1 *Statistical Account* Vol VI Ayrshire (Lochwinnoch)
2 *Statistical Account* Vol VII Lanarkshire and Renfrewshire (East Kilbride)
3 *Statistical Account* Vol XII North and West Perthshire (Blackford)
4 *Statistical Account* Vol XII North and West Perthshire (Little Dunkeld)
5 Thomas Pennant *A Tour in Scotland and Voyage to the Hebrides* (London 1772)
6 Osgood H Mackenzie *A Hundred Years in the Highlands* (Edward Arnold 1924)
7 *Statistical Account* Vol XII North and West Perthshire (Dunkeld and Dowally)

8   *Statistical Account* Vol VII Lanarkshire and Renfrewshire (Glasford)
9   *Statistical Account* Vol XII North and West Perthshire (Clunie)

Chapter 3

1   *Statistical Account* Vol XII North and West Perthshire (Fortingall)
2   Elizabeth Grant *Memoirs of a Highland Lady 1797–1827* (John Murray, London 1898)
3   *Statistical Account* Vol XII North and West Perthshire (Clunie)
4   James Boswell *Journal of a Tour to the Hebrides* (London 1773)
5   Edward Burt *Letters from a Gentleman in the North of Scotland* (London 1754)
6   Henry G Graham *The Social Life of Scotland in the Eighteenth Century* (Adam and Charles Black, London 1899)
7   Sir John Sinclair, *Appendix to the General Report for Scotland 1814* (David Willison, Edinburgh)
8   Henry G Graham op. cit.
9   Sir Walter Scott *Guy Mannering* (Edinburgh 1815)
10 Henry G Graham op. cit.
11 Sir Walter Scott op. cit.
12 Elizabeth Grant op. cit.
13 Henry G Graham op. cit.
14 Dr Samuel Johnson *A Journey to the Western Isles of Scotland* (London 1773)
15 James Boswell op. cit.
16 Henry G Graham op. cit.
17 Dr John Macculloch *The Highlands and Western Isles of Scotland* (London 1824)
18 Dorothy Wordsworth *Recollections of a Tour made in Scotland in AD 1803* (London 1804)
19 Henry G Graham op. cit.
20 Dean Edward Ramsay *Reminiscences of Scottish Life and Character* (Edinburgh 1857)
21 Ochtertyre House Booke of Accomps, 1737–1739

Chapter 4

1   Dr Samuel Johnson *A Journey to the Western Isles of Scotland* (London 1773)
2   William Cramond, *The Records of Elgin,* 1234–1800 (New Spalding Club, Aberdeen 1903)
3   James Boswell *Journal of a Tour to the Hebrides* (London 1773)
4   Edward Burt *Letters from a Gentleman in the North of Scotland* (London 1754).
5   *Statistical Account* Vol XII North and West Perthshire (Bendothy)
6   David Kerr Cameron *The Ballad and the Plough* (Futura 1979)
7   Dr Samuel Johnson op. cit.

8 *Statistical Account* Vol XII North and West Perthshire (Callander)
9 Alexander Fenton 'Traditional Elements in the Diet of the Northern Isles of Scotland', *Shetland Times,* 1976
10 Nancy Watt 'Mary Stewart of Glen Tarken'. Unpublished MS.
11 *Statistical Account* Vol XII North and West Perthshire (Bendothy)
12 Thomas Pennant *A Tour in Scotland and Voyage to the Hebrides* (London 1772)
13 Martin Martin *A Description of the Western Isles of Scotland* (Eneas Mackay 1934)
14 Tom Steel *The Life and Death of St Kilda* (National Trust for Scotland, Edinburgh 1965)
15 John Taylor *The Pennyless Pilgrimage* (London 1618)
16 Dr Samuel Johnson op. cit.
17 James Boswell op. cit.
18 Osgood H Mackenzie *A Hundred Years in the Highlands* (Edward Arnold 1924)
19 James Logan, *The Scottish Gael* (James Donald 1831)
20 Thomas Newte *A Tour in England and Scotland performed in 1785* (London 1798)
21 Alexander Fenton *Scottish Country Life* (John Donald 1974).
22 The Ochertyre House Book of Accomps, 1737–1739
23 James Logan op. cit.
24 Thomas Pennant op. cit.
25 Edward Burt op. cit.
26 *Statistical Account* Vol VII Lanarkshire and Renfrewshire (Kilbarchan)
27 *Statistical Account* Vol VII Lanarkshire and Renfrewshire (Cambuslang)
28 *Statistical Account* Vol XII North and West Perthshire (Crieff)
29 Thomas Pennant op. cit.
30 Sir Walter Scott *Waverley* (Edinburgh 1814)
31 Edward Burt op. cit.
32 Thomas Pennant op. cit.
33 *Statistical Account* Vol XII North and West Perthshire (Dunkeld and Dowally)
34 James Boswell op. cit.
35 F Marian McNeill *The Scots Kitchen* (Blackie 1929)
36 Dr Samuel Johnson op. cit.
37 *Statistical Account* Vol VII Lanarkshire and Renfrewshire (Symington)
38 *Statistical Account* Vol XII North and West Perthshire (Bendothy)
39 *Statistical Account* Vol VII Lanarkshire and Renfrewshire (Cadder)
40 James T Calder *Sketch of the Civil and Traditional History of Caithness* (Wick 1887)
41 Osgood H Mackenzie op. cit.
42 Dr Samuel Johnson op. cit.
43 *Statistical Account* Vol XII North and West Perthshire (Dunkeld and Dowally).
44 Osgood H Mackenzie op. cit.

45 *Statistical Account* Vol VII Lanarkshire and Renfrewshire (Carluke)
46 *Statistical Account* Vol VII Lanarkshire and Renfrewshire (Hamilton)
47 *Statistical Account* Vol VII Lanarkshire and Renfrewshire (Carstairs)
48 Edward Burt op. cit.
49 Alexander Carmichael (ed) *Carmina Gadelica*
50 Martin Martin op. cit.
51 *Statistical Account* Vol XII North and West Perthshire (Blackford)
52 *Statistical Account* Vol XI South and East Perthshire and Kinross-shire (Arngask)
53 *Statistical Account* Vol VII Lanarkshire and Renfrewshire (Hamilton)
54 Dr James Lind *A Treatise of the Scurvy* (London 1753)
55 Douglas Guthrie *A History of Medicine* (Nelson 1945)
56 Henry G Graham op. cit.
57 *Statistical Account* Vol VII Lanarkshire and Renfrewshire (Glasgow)
58 *Statistical Account* Vol VII Lanarkshire and Renfrewshire (Carnwath)
59 Dr Samuel Johnson op. cit.
60 Elizabeth Grant op. cit.
61 James Boswell op. cit.
62 Eric Linklater *The Prince in the Heather* (Hodder and Stoughton 1965)
63 Martin Martin op. cit.
64 Henry G Graham op. cit.
65 *Statistical Account* Vol XII North and West Perthshire (Crieff)
66 *Statistical Account* Vol XII North and West Perthshire (Lecropt)

Chapter 5

1 Robert Louis Stevenson *Travels with a Donkey in the Cevennes* (Edinburgh 1879)
2 Edward Burt *Letters from a Gentleman in the North of Scotland* (London 1754)
3 Elizabeth Haldane *The Scotland of our Fathers* (Glasgow University Press 1933)
4 Edward Burt op. cit.
5 Faujas de St Fond *Tour in Scotland 1784* (1797)
6 Edward Burt op. cit.
7 John Wesley *Journal 1761*
8 John V Taylor *Enough is Enough* (SCM Press 1975)

Chapter 6

1 William Ferguson *Scotland, 1689 to the Present* (Oliver and Boyd 1968)
2 Daniel Defoe *A Tour through the whole Island of Great Britain* (London 1727)
3 *Statistical Account* Vol VII Lanarkshire and Renfrewshire (Glasgow)
4 *Statistical Account* Vol VII Lanarkshire and Renfrewshire (Hamilton)

5 *Statistical Account* Vol XII North and West Perthshire (Moulin)
6 *Statistical Account* Vol VII Lanarkshire and Renfrewshire (Lanark)
7 Henry G Graham *The Social Life of Scotland in the Eighteenth Century* (Adam and Charles Black, London 1899)
8 *Statistical Account* Vol XII North and West Perthshire (Callander)
9 Elizabeth Haldane *The Scotland of our Fathers* (Glasgow University Press 1933)
10 *New Statistical Account* (Edinburgh)
11 *New Statistical Account* (Dundee)
12 Elizabeth Haldane op. cit.
13 *New Statistical Account* (Leith)
14 Elizabeth Haldane op. cit.

Chapter 7

1 Edwin Muir *Scottish Journey* (Mainstream, Edinburgh 1935)
2 J C Drummond and A Wilbraham *The Englishman's Food* (Jonathan Cape 1938)
3 F G Hopkins 'The Analyst and the Medical Man' *The Analyst, 31,* p 385 (1906)
4 Noreen Branson *Britain in the Nineteen Twenties* (Weidenfeld and Nicolson 1975)
5 Report No 101 (Medical Research Council 1925)

Chapter 8

1 Sir John Boyd Orr *Food, Health and Income* (Macmillan 1936)
2 Sir Robert McCarrison *Nutrition and Health* (Faber 1953)
3 A H Kitchin and R Passmore *The Scotsman's Food* (E and S Livingstone 1949)
4 Dr John V G A Durnin, article in *Glasgow Herald* May 1972
5 E McIntyre, article in *Glasgow Herald* (date unknown)
6 D P Burkitt 'Fibre-depleted Carbohydrates and Disease', Community Health, *(Journal)* 1975
7 K W Heaton 'Are we getting too much out of food? *Journal of Human Nutrition*, 1973 Vol 27, p 170
8 *British Medical Journal* 'Food and Fibre', 1977, Vol 2, p 418

Chapter 9

1 Paul E Stemann *Across the Highlands with Sweetheart* (Hale 1970)
2 Molly Weir *Shoes were for Sunday* (Pan Books 1970)
3 Dorothy Hollingsworth 'A National Nutrition Policy: Can we devise one?' *Journal of Human Nutrition,* 1979 Vol 33, p. 211
4 C J Robbins (ed) 'Food, Health and Farming: Reports of panels on the implications for UK agriculture?' *Centre for Agricultural Strategy paper,* 7 November 1978.
5 Dr W W Yellowlees 'Ill Fares the Land', James Mackenzie Memorial Lecture, 1978

Chapter 10

1 Ritchie Calder *Common Sense about a Starving World* (Gollancz 1962)
2 Susan George *How the Other Half Dies* (Pelican Books 1976)
3 Ritchie Calder op. cit.
4 *North/South: A Programme for Survival* (Pan Books 1979)
5 E F Schumacher *Small is Beautiful (Economics as if People Mattered)* (Harper and Row 1973)
6 George Hoffman 'Tear Times' (1983)
7 Leading article, 'Sensible Eating' *British Medical Journal* 1977 Vol 2, p 80
8 Claude Aubert 'A Food Policy for the Third World' *Nutrition and Health,* 1983 Vol II, No. 1

Chapter 11

1 John Hawthorn *Is Good Food a Fad?* Van den Bergh Series No 5
2 Alan Harrison 'Food Education and School Meals: are they on Separate Tables? *Nutrition and Food Science,* Jan/Feb 1983
3 'National Food Policy in the UK' (Report), Centre for Agricultural Strategy, 1979
4 Eating for Health (DHSS Report) HMSO 1978
5 A H Kitchin and R Passmore *The Scotsman's Food* (E and S Livingstone 1949)
6 Yehudi Menuhin *Unfinished Journey* (Futura 1978)
7 Susan George *How the Other Half Dies* (Pelican Books 1976)
8 Dr W W Yellowlees 'Ill Fares the Land' James Mackenzie Memorial Lecture, 1978
9 Martin Martin *A Description of the Western Isles of Scotland* (Eneas Mackay 1934)
10 James Logan *The Scottish Gael* (John Donald 1831)
11 John V Taylor *Enough is Enough* (SCM Press 1975)
12 Erik Dammann *The Future in our Hands* (Pergamon Press 1979)

BIBLIOGRAPHY

SOCIAL HISTORY AND GENERAL INTEREST

Boswell, James *Journal of a Tour to the Hebrides with Samuel Johnson* (London 1773)

Branson, Noreen *Britain in the Nineteen Twenties* (Weidenfeld & Nicolson 1975)

Burt, Capt Edward *Letters from a Gentleman in the North of Scotland* (London 1754)

Calder, James T *Sketch of the Civil and Traditional History of Caithness* (Wick 1887)

Cameron, David Kerr *The Ballad and the Plough* (Futura 1979)

Campbell, R H *Scotland since 1707* (Basil Blackwell 1965)

Campbell, R H and Dow, J B A *Source Book of Scottish Economic and Social History* (Blackwell, Edinburgh 1968)

Chambers, Robert *Domestic Annals of Scotland* (Edinburgh 1885)

Chitnis, Anand *The Scottish Enlightenment* (Croom Helm, London, 1976)

Daiches, David *Glasgow* (Andre Deutsch 1977)

Defoe, Daniel *A Tour Through the Whole Island of Great Britain* (1727)

Donaldson, Gordon *Scotland: The Shaping of a Nation* (David & Charles 1974)

Fenton, Alexander *Scottish Country Life* (John Donald 1974)

_____ 'Traditional Elements in the Diet of the Northern Isles of Scotland' (Shetland Times 1976)

Ferguson, William *Scotland, 1689 to the Present* (Oliver & Boyd 1968)

Graham, Henry G *The Social Life of Scotland in the 18th Century* (Adam & Chas Black, London 1899)

Grant, Elizabeth *Memoirs of a Highland Lady 1797–1827* (John Murray, London 1898)

Grant, I F *Highland Folk Ways* (Routledge & Kegan Paul 1961)

_____ *Every-day Life on an Old Highland Farm* (Shepheard-Walwyn 1924)

Haldane, A R B *The Drove Roads of Scotland* (Nelson 1952)

Haldane, E *The Scotland of our Fathers* (University Press, Glasgow 1933)

Hibben, Frank C *Prehistoric Man in Europe* (Constable, London 1959)

Johnson, Dr Samuel *A Journey to the Western Isles of Scotland* (1773)

Lethbridge, T C *The Painted Men* (Andrew Melrose, London 1954)

Linklater, Eric *The Prince in the Heather* (Hodder & Stoughton, 1965)

Logan, James *The Scottish Gael* (John Donald 1831)

Mackie, J D *A History of Scotland* (Penguin Books 1964)
Martin Martin *A Description of the Western Isles of Scotland* (circa 1695) (Eneas Mackay, Stirling 1934)
Marwick, Arthur *Women at War 1914–1918* (Fontana 1977)
Mavor, William (ed) *The British Tourists (Celebrated Tours in the British Islands)* (1798)
Menuhin, Yehudi *Unfinished Journey* (Futura 1978)
Muir, Edwin *Scottish Journey* (Mainstream Publishing, Edinburgh 1935)
Mackenzie, Osgood H *A Hundred Years in the Highlands* (Edward Arnold 1924)
Newte, Thomas *Prospects and Observations on a Tour of England & Scotland, 1791*
Pennant, Thomas *A Tour in Scotland and Voyage to the Hebrides* (1772)
Piggott, Stuart and Henderson, Keith *Scotland Before History* (Nelson 1958)
Ramsay, Dean Edward, *Reminiscences of Scottish Life and Character*(Edinburgh 1857)
Sinclair, Sir John *Appendix to the General Report of Scotland, 1814* David Willison Edinburgh)
_____ *Analysis of the Statistical Account* (Edinburgh 1831)
Smout, T C *A History of the Scottish People 1560–1830* (Collins 1969)
Steel, Tom *The Life and Death of St. Kilda* (National Trust for Scotland 1965)
Stemann, Paul E, *Across the Highlands with Sweetheart* (Hale 1970)
Stevenson, R L *Travels with a Donkey in the Cevennes* (1879)
Thomson, George Malcolm *Scotland, That Distressed Area* (Porpoise Press, Edinburgh 1935)
Weir, Molly *Shoes Were for Sunday* (Pan Books 1970)
Wesley, John *Journal* (visited Scotland 1761–2)
Wordsworth, Dorothy *Recollections of a Tour Made in Scotland in AD 1803* (London 1804)

FOOD, NUTRITION, MEDICINE

Boyd Orr, Sir John *Food, Health and Income* (Macmillan 1936)
Cleave, T L *The Saccharine Disease* (John Wright, Bristol, 1974)
Davidson, S, Passmore, R, Brock, J F and Truswell, A S *Human Nutrition and Dietetics,* 6th ed, (Churchill Livingstone 1975)
Drummond, J C and Wilbraham, A *The Englishman's Food* (Jonathan Cape 1938)
Guthrie, Douglas *A History of Medicine* (Nelson 1945)
Kitchin, A H and Passmore, R *The Scotsman's Food* (E & S Livingstone 1949)
Lind, J *A Treatise of the Scurvy* (London 1753, reprinted EUP 1953)
McCance, R A and Widdowson, E M *The Composition of Foods* (HMSO London, 1960)
McCarrison, R *Nutrition and Health* (Faber & Faber 1953)
MacClure, Victor *Scotland's Inner Man* George Routledge & Sons 1935)

McCallum, E V *A History of Nutrition* Massachusetts, 1957)
McNeill, F Marian *The Scots Kitchen* (Blackie 1929)
Ochtertyre House Booke of Accomps (1737–9)
Tannahill, R *Food in History* (Paladin 1975)

Dietary Calculations from: *The Composition of Foods*. R A McCance and
    E M Widdowson HMSO, London 1960)

WORLD DEVELOPMENT

Calder, Ritchie, *Common Sense About a Starving World* (Victor Gollancz
    1962)
George, Susan *How The Other Half Dies* (*The Real Reasons for World
    Hunger*) (Pelican Books 1976)
_____ *Feeding the Few*: *Corporate Control of Food* (Institute for Policy
    Studies 1979)
Lappé, Frances Moore and Collins, Joseph *World Hunger: Ten Myths*
    (Institute for Food & Development Policy 1979)
Lean, Geoffrey *Rich World, Poor World* (Allen & Unwin 1980)
Schumacher, E F *Small is Beautiful (Economics as if People Mattered)*
    (Harper & Row 1973)
Sider, Ronald *Rich Christians in an Age of Hunger* (Hodder & Stoughton
    1977)
Tanner, John *A New Deal for the Poor* (World Development Movement
    1976)
Taylor, John V *Enough is Enough* (SCM Press 1975)

PAPERS AND REPORTS

Baker, Paul *It's Up To Us* (Scottish Education & Action for Development
    1980)
DHSS *Eating for Health* (HMSO 1978)
_____ *Nutrition Education* (HMSO)
FAO Report *World Food Day* (1981)
Food First Resource Guide (Institute for Food & Development Policy
    1979)
National Food Policy in the UK (Centre for Agricultural Strategy 1979)
Food, Health & Farming (Centre for Agricultural Strategy 1978)
North/South: A Programme for Survival (Pan Books 1979)
The Statistical Account of Scotland (various volumes) 1791–9
The New Statistical Account of Scotland (various volumes) 1835–45
Yellowlees, W W *Ill Fares the Land* James Mackenzie Memorial Lecture
    1978
Wynn, Arthur *Malnutrition Around Conception as a Cause of Congenital
    Malformation and other Handicaps* (Paper presented at the
    McCarrison Society Scottish Group Conference 1982)
MRC Report No 101 *The Health of Scottish Children*

ARTICLES

British Medical Journal

Year	Vol	Page		
1976	I	1346	Rickets in Asian Immigrants	Dunnigan, McIntosh, Ford
1977	I	341	Who is at risk of a Coronary?	Khosla, Newcombe, Campbell
1977	I	867	Dietary recommendations for the community towards the postponement of coronary heart disease	Shaper, Marr
1977	I	1115	How dangerous is obesity?	Leading article
1977	II	80	Sensible eating	
1977	II	418	Food and fibre	
1979	I	173	Eats and atheroma: an inquest	McMichael
1979	I	527	Prescription for a better British diet	Passmore, Hollingsworth, Robertson
1979	II	1541	Dietary fibre and blood pressure	Wright, Burstyn, Gibney
1980	280	177	Dietary prevention of ischaemic heart disease—A policy for the eighties	Lewis
1980	280	1396	Effects of high dietary sugar	Yudkin, Kang, Bruckdorfer
1982	285	1321	Dietary Advice	Fowler

Journal of Human Nutrition

1973	27	170	Are we getting too much out of food?	Heaton
1974	29	337	The livestock of Great Britain as food producers	Holmes
1976	30	9	Value of traditional practices in nutrition education	Church, Doughty
1978	32	439	Unconventional sources of protein	Scrimgeour
1979	33	211	A national nutrition policy: can we devise one?	Hollingsworth
1979	33	57	A prudent diet for the nation	Mann
1980	34	161	Nutritional labelling	Allen

Soil, Food & Health in a Changing World (1980)

			Health and agricultural policies in conflict	Robbins
			Sir Robert McCarrison: his relevance today	Yellowlees

Community Health Journal

| 1975 6, 4 | 190 | Fibre–depleted carbohydrates and disease | Burkitt |

Scottish Geographical Magazine

| 1977 | April | Fisheries in Scotland in the 16th, 17th & 18th centuries | Coull |

Nutrition and Food Science

| 1983 | January February | Food education and school meals: are they on separate tables? | Harrison |

Getting The Most out of Food

Van den Bergh's—
Series No. 5   Is good food a fad?   Hawthorn

Nutrition and Health

Vol. 2, No. 1   A food policy for the Third
World   Aubert
Vol. 2, No. 2   The prevention of neural
tube
defects: a public health
approach   St George
Vol. 2, No. 3/4 Dietary approaches to the
prevention of neural tube
defects   Lawrence

INDEX